Central and South American Medical Schools – Caribbean Region

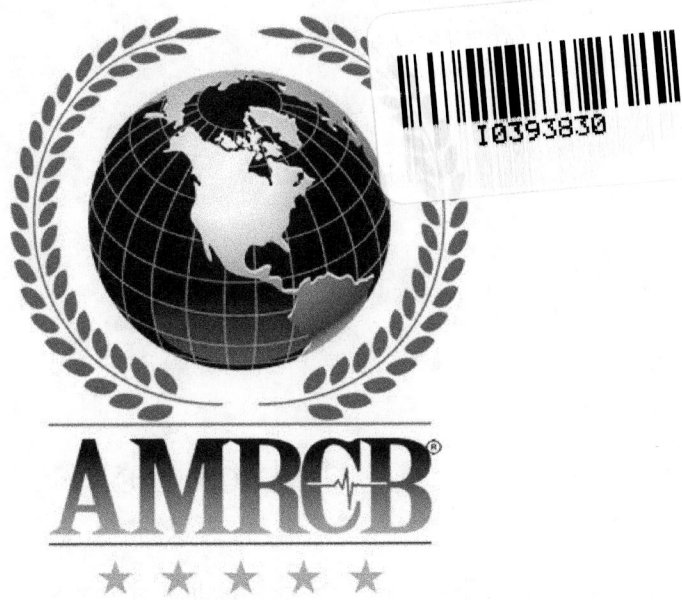

Copyright © 2015 American Medical Residency Certification Board

All rights reserved.

ISBN-13:978-1505589931

ISBN-10: 1505589932

CreateSpace Independent Publishing Platform, North Charleston, SC

All materials subject to these copyrights may be photocopied for the purpose of nonprofit, scientific, or educational advancement.

Suggested Citation
Central and South American Medical Schools (Caribbean Region) based on a U.S. Curriculum - American Medical Residency Certification Board®, 2015

DEDICATION

This book is dedicated to potential medical school students across the globe. While the aim of this book is to describe Central and South American Schools in the Caribbean region that follow the North American educational model for students who desire to practice medicine in the United States, we hope that students across the international community will find this reference a useful tool. The AMRCB® wishes all students success in their chosen fields.

ADDITIONAL AMRCB® PUBLICATIONS

Caribbean Medical Schools Based on a U.S. Curriculum – Greater and Lesser Antilles. American Medical Residency Certification Board®, 2014. ISBN-13: 978-1500419042, ISBN-10: 1500419044

Passing the AMRCB® Certification Conference. American Medical Residency Certification Board®, 2015 – ISBN-13: 978-150558993,1 ISBN-10:1505589932

Irish Medical Schools – Based on a U.S. Curriculum. American Medical Residency Certification Board®, 2015. Expected Publication in summer 2015

Canadian Medical Schools. American Medical Residency Certification Board®, 2015. ISBN-13: 978-1507817177 ISBN-10:1507817179

CONTENTS

	Forward	v
1	Caribbean Medical Schools	Pg #1
2	Licensure	Pg #7
3	The Application Process	Pg #31
4	The Interview	Pg #43
5	Residency	Pg #53
6	IMG Data	Pg #61
7	Financial Aid	Pg #81
8	The Islands	Pg #96
9	The Schools	Pg #103

Central and South American Medical Schools – Caribbean Region

ACKNOWLEDGMENTS

Steven W. Powell, MD, MPH, CPE, FAPA - Primary Author

Adnan Khan, MD

Dennis Sehgal, MD - Forward

FORWARD

Dear Future Physician,

I would like to start off by saying thank you for being ambitious and choosing medicine as your desired profession. It takes unique individuals with dynamic mindsets to make such a decision, thus you will become an essential and key addition to the healthcare system. Studying to become a doctor of medicine in the Caribbean region allows you to acquire some of the finest education that is available. The standard is set so that learning in the Caribbean region is equivalent to North American, European, and other educational systems throughout the world. This is attested to by the phenomenal programs and professors that are selected from many different countries that provide outstanding medical education to the students that choose a Caribbean education.

There is no place like the Caribbean region to begin such a journey. To most people, these areas are known as vacation destinations. You will have the benefit of calling places like Turks and Caicos your "home" for a period of time. The natural habitat is beautiful as the mountain peaks touch down to sandy beaches creating a scenic environment that is truly peaceful. A variety of activities allow interests of any individual to be enjoyed. Whether you like jet skiing, playing beach volleyball, riding scooters, reading a book by the pool, or taking in other aspects of the culture, you will surely be pleased.

Of course becoming a physician is not as easy as lying on the beach and getting a tan in the year-round beautiful sunny weather. Medical school does require endless effort and dedication. Fulfilling your dream to care for people will require sacrifice. Studying in the Caribbean allows opportunity to gain unfamiliar experiences and being away from home creates the ability to grow as an individual who can ultimately become an independent professional. It is equally as important to make progress as a human being alongside your education to become a complete, competent medical caregiver.

Being someone who has completed this journey, I can wholeheartedly say that I would not trade my background for any alternative. Living around those who are local to the islands and learning the ways of life, without all of the modern technology I was used to, truly grew on me. Although most normal amenities are available, native life created awareness that living modestly can be very sensible and enjoyable. I was able to appreciate the natural environment and able to live the relaxed lifestyle that was portrayed, while successfully excelling through medical school.

Don't get me wrong. As excited I was about all of the potential luxuries before going, it wasn't exactly as advertised. Yes - the mountains, the beaches, and all of the beauty of the region is there during your down time; but leaving home had its challenges. It was hard to leave friends, family, and the life that I was accustomed to. However, after realizing that everyone else was doing the same with a similar mindset; adjusting to the challenges became effortless. We grew together and created new friendships. Many of us are still in touch today and some of us even work together. Not only did we rely on each other, but we relied on members of the community, professors, and other staff as well to provide support and guidance though our struggles.

Most people do not have the opportunity, or even the thought, of leaving their comfort zone. Life by many is thought of as growing up, becoming educated, and ultimately working in one place. Although there is nothing wrong with that mindset, and even if the ultimate goal is to work and live where you grew up; having the ability to say that you went to school on an island and completed your clinical clerkships in different cities throughout North America or globally is an amazing privilege. This truly sets you apart from the mundane path that many have taken in life.

We truly believe that understanding, education, and training from Central or South American medical schools in the Caribbean region will create an unmatched foundation for you as a person and as a healthcare provider. These experiences will allow you to enjoy diverse cultures from a different point of view. After taking part in local communities and healthcare systems, your ability to relate, teach, and innovate at any level of medicine in any environment will be admired by your supervisors, your colleagues, and most importantly your patients!

If you do choose the Caribbean region as your route to complete your passion and goals, make it a priority to take it all in. Fulfill all your scholarly requirements in an exceptional manner but also venture out and enjoy the many attributes the region has to offer.

On your voyage to becoming a physician, we extend to you our best wishes!

Sincerely,

Dennis Sehgal, MD
AMRCB® Canadian Physician Advisor

INTRODUCTION

International medical schools that base their educational curriculum on the model used by United States and provide instruction in English are listed below. Medical school locations are listed based on physiographic location and divided by those listed in this publication and those in the Greater and Lesser Antilles described in the AMRCB® Caribbean Medical School publication. Islands that lie on the South American geologic shelf are listed in the Central and South American publication and include Aruba, Bonaire, Curacao, and Trinidad and Tobago. Other medical schools may exist in these areas as well but are not listed in this publication if instruction is not in English or if the educational curriculum does not follow U.S. standards.

Medical schools listed in this publication include:

CENTRAL AND SOUTH AMERICA
(Caribbean Region)

CENTRAL AMERICA

Belize: pg. #110

- American Global University School of Medicine
- Avicina Medical Academy
- Central America Health Sciences University Belize Medical College
- Grace University School of Medicine
- Hope University School of Medicine
- InterAmerican Medical University
- Medical University of the Americas
- St. Luke's University School of Medicine
- St. Matthew's University School of Medicine
- Washington University of Health and Sciences

Panama: pg. #190

- Columbus University School of Medicine and Health Sciences

SOUTH AMERICA
Aruba: pg. #204

- Aureus University School of Medicine
- Xavier University School of Medicine

Bonaire: pg. #224

- St. James School of Medicine – Bonaire

Curacao: pg. #236

- Avalon University School of Medicine
- Caribbean Medical University School of Medicine
- St. Martinus University Faculty of Medicine

Guyana: pg. #272

- American International School of Medicine
- GreenHeart Medical University School of Medicine
- Texila American University College of Medicine
- University of Guyana Faculty of Health Sciences

Trinidad and Tobago: pg. #314

- University of the West Indies Faculty of Medicine - St. Augustine

The following medical schools are described in the AMRCB® publication entitled: Caribbean Medical Schools – Greater and Lesser Antilles - Based on a U.S. Curriculum – The Complete Guide to Medical Schools, Acceptance Criteria, and International Life. The third edition was released in 2014, ISBN 978-1500419042

Anguilla:

- Saint James School of Medicine – Anguilla

Antigua and Barbuda:

- American University of Antigua College of Medicine
- University of Health Sciences Antigua School of Medicine

Barbados:

- American University of Barbados School of Medicine
- University of the West Indies - Barbados Faculty of Medical Sciences

Cayman Islands:

- St. Matthew's University School of Medicine

Dominica:

- All Saints University School of Medicine
- Ross University School of Medicine

Dominican Republic:

- Universidad Iberoamericana (UNIBE) School of Medicine

Grenada:

- St. George's University School of Medicine

Jamaica:

- All American Institute of Medical Sciences
- University of the West Indies Faculty of Medical Sciences - Kingstown

Montserrat:

- Seoul Central College of Medicine
- University of Science, Arts, & Technology (USAT) Faculty of Medicine
- Vanguard University School of Medicine

Saba:

- Saba University School of Medicine

Saint Kitts and Nevis:

- Burnett International University School of Medicine and Health Sciences
- Grace University School of Medicine
- International University of the Health Sciences
- Medical University of the Americas
- Milik University
- Saint Theresa's Medical University
- University of Medicine and Health Sciences
- Windsor University School of Medicine

Saint Lucia:

- American International Medical University School of Medicine
- Atlantic University School of Medicine
- College of Medicine and Health Sciences
- Destiny University School of Medicine and Health Sciences
- International American University College of Medicine
- Spartan Health Sciences University School of Medicine
- St. Helen University School of Medicine
- St. Mary's School of Medicine
- Washington Medical Sciences Institute

Saint Martin:

- American University of the Caribbean School of Medicine
- University of Sint Eustatius School of Medicine

Saint Vincent and the Grenadines:

- All Saints University College of Medicine
- American University of St. Vincent School of Medicine
- Kingstown Medical College
- Saint James School of Medicine - St. Vincent and the Grenadines
- Trinity School of Medicine

Chapter 1
Central and South American Medical Schools

The medical schools located throughout Central and South America provides an opportunity for countless students to obtain their medical degrees. If a prospective student harbors the idea that attending medical school in Central and South America will be an adventure, then they will be able to make the most of the experience. Each school, as well as the entire Central and South America region, offer many positive experiences that would not be available in other parts of the world. Many students have also perceived negative aspects as well. Living in Central and South America and obtaining an education from a school other than one in the United States can be challenging and may lead to many frustrating experiences, particularly for those who are U.S. citizens and desire to practice medicine in the United States upon graduation.

It is important to understand that Central and South America medical schools are just one option to receive a medical education. Other educational options across the globe are available to medical students from the U.S. and other countries who want to obtain a medical education. This book is written from the perspective of U.S. citizens who are looking to obtain a medical education outside of the U.S. educational system. What can be difficult with medical school for U.S. citizens that are located in areas other than the Caribbean region is that there is often varied educational content, and the limited exposure to the U.S. healthcare system can make acceptance into a U.S. medical residency and/or the eventual practice of medicine inside the United States more difficult.

PROS

The majority of Central and South America medical schools offer a split campus program designed so that the first two basic science years are completed in the Americas and the last two clinical years are completed at affiliated hospitals in the United States or at other locations across the globe. Not every student will get to spend their clinical rotation years in the United States as many schools offer these spots only to the most competitive applicants. Completing the clinical years in the United States will give Caribbean and Central and South America graduates an edge when it comes to obtaining a U.S. residency position. Most other international medical schools throughout Mexico, Europe, and other locales are not able to offer these same benefits.

Many Central and South America medical schools offer a curriculum that is modeled after programs in the United States. The education and course content is often identical to the finest United States medical schools. Except for the rare instance in primarily Spanish speaking countries, all textbooks are in English and all courses are taught in English allowing for better preparation for the licensing exams than may be available at other international medical schools. Note taking services are, however, generally not available for students as they are in the United States. The medical and basic science faculties at these schools are M.D.'s, D.O.'s, and Ph.D.'s and offer a broad exposure to cultures from different parts of the world. Some of the schools will also allow the completion of a M.D. degree in an accelerated manner in less than four calendar years which is not available with medical schools located within the United States.

Most Central and South America schools have three entering classes per year, and it is much easier to get accepted than it is at United States medical schools. Classes will generally start in January, May, and September for some schools and only in January and September for others. This allows for two to three times as many students to be accepted each year as would normally be accepted with only one starting class each year in the United States. The most popular starting class application is for the classes that begin in September. This class will often fill up the earliest at each school resulting in last minute applications from those not accepted at United States schools being denied for this class. Almost every school has a system in place that will allow those not accepted in the September class to be offered a spot in the January class or other future classes. January and May classes are often not completely filled, and spots are consistently available in these classes. It is important for a student who wants to begin classes in September to apply very early in the academic year.

Most Central and South America medical schools offer financial aid and loan programs that are similar to those in the United States. These aid programs are set up primarily for United States and Canadian citizens and may be more difficult to obtain for those without citizenship in these countries. The United States has made available over $20 million in financial aid for qualified students attending many foreign medical schools. Other loans may be available for international students. The programs offered at most schools include Canadian Student Loans, Subsidized and Unsubsidized Federal Stafford Loans, the International Health Education Loan Program (TERI), Veterans benefits, as well as many various private scholarships. Each school is different and the loans that are available and offered can change. Recently, one school lost their ability to offer Stafford loans for a year just because they missed the mailing deadline for recertification.

Bottom line - beware and be prepared.

CONS

Many challenges are present for those who choose to attend Central and South America medical schools. As an international medical student, it will be harder to obtain a medical internship and residency, gain licensure, and ultimately practice medicine in the United States. Hard work and diligence can, however, accomplish this. It will be necessary to do much better than the average United States graduate on each step of the licensing exams, and additional tests and evaluation steps will often be required. If a student is fully prepared for these circumstances, they can succeed.

A student that is able to obtain a position in the United States for clinical rotations will have to travel frequently. Most clinical rotations are offered in different states for different time periods. This variation results in travel from state to state and difficulty at times finding housing. It is not uncommon to wait for weeks between each clinical rotation. Delays may occur while rotations open up and may also occur if the school loses clinical contracts. Students with nightmare stories about being stuck for weeks and months because of unforeseen problems are not impossible to find. The schools work hard to avoid this, but it can, and does, happen.

The success rates for Central and South America graduates can be less than impressive. Only 64% of students who seek a medical degree from Central and South America will pass the first step of the licensing exam on their first try. Many medical schools in the Central and South America will advertise very high USMLE® pass rates, but they often have internal USMLE® practice testing that prohibits students from taking the actual USMLE® until they achieve a certain percentage on the practice exam. This can result in an inflated rate of actual USMLE® performance as many students never progress to the point of being able to actually sit for the exam. In addition, only one-third of the students will graduate on time. Another one-third will graduate late, and the other third will never realize their dream of becoming a physician. A prospective student must be aware of, and understand, these statistics. The attrition rate at United States schools is less than 2% while it is 20-30% for Central and South American medical schools. These statistics can be interpreted in several ways. Most importantly is the fact that these are students who are given a chance to pursue their dream of practicing medicine. Failures will occur, but the students at least had the chance. A student must enter with the mindset that they will succeed and will be willing to work hard to achieve their goals.

The facilities at some Central and South America schools are less than pristine. Some schools have new facilities that are air-conditioned, hurricane proof, and technologically advanced. However, other medical schools may have small, non-air-conditioned facilities with little technology and resources. Some schools have student housing but many do not. It is very important that a prospective student investigates any schools to which they are applying and, if possible, personally visit the school prior to accepting a place in the matriculating class. A few schools will require a personal interview, but most are held over the phone or as regional interviews. This varies from school to school and is often decided on an individual basis. Again, if at all possible, personally visit the school!

Chapter 2
Licensure

Physicians trained in Central and South America are required to navigate two additional tests to gain licensure in the United States compared with their United States counterparts. Central and South America graduates had previously been required to pass a third additional test as well until 2005 when United States students were required to take the Clinical Skills Assessment in order to practice medicine. Previously this test was only required of international graduates. The Educational Commission for Foreign Medical Graduates (ECFMG®) English Proficiency test is required for international graduates while not for U.S. graduates. This test is designed to test the abilities and English proficiency of future medical professionals. In addition, certification by the American Medical Residency Certification Board (AMRCB®) is utilized by many international graduates to demonstrate a sign of excellence and readiness to enter a U.S. medical internship or residency position. AMRCB® certification remains voluntary at the time of this publication.

The required steps to practice medicine within the United States are as follows:

    Step 1: USMLE® Step 1

    Step 2: USMLE® Step 2 CS and Step 2 CK

    Step 3: ECFMG® Certification

Step 4: AMRCB® Certification (Discretionary)

Step 5: Acceptance, and eventual completion, of a United States medical residency

Step 6: USMLE® Step 3

USMLE®

The United States Medical Licensing Exam (USMLE®) is a standardized test that is designed to provide a common evaluation system for students regardless of where they received their medical education. The test is a multiple choice exam and is divided into three steps that must be taken and passed by anyone desiring to practice medicine in the United States. In 1999, Step 1 and Step 2 were converted from a paper format to a computer-based format thus paper administrations of Step 1 and Step 2 are no longer available. The computer-based administrations of Step 1 and Step 2 are offered continuously at over 500 test centers worldwide.

Step 1 is concerned with the basic medical sciences and assesses if a student can apply the understanding and knowledge of key concepts of the basic biomedical science. The mechanisms and principles of health, disease, and modes of therapy are assessed. Step 1 is the test used to demonstrate mastery of the basic sciences and that students have a basic foundation of this knowledge. Step 1 is usually taken at the end of the second year between the basic and clinical science years. The test is given over one day and consists of 322 multiple-choice questions and is divided into 7 blocks of 46 questions. It is a requirement by most schools that Step 1 is passed prior to beginning study of the clinical sciences. The current minimum passing score has been raised to 192, and has been raised several times over the last 2 decades.

USMLE® Step 2 Clinical Knowledge (CK) concentrates on the clinical sciences. This step assesses if a student can apply the medical knowledge and understanding of the clinical sciences, which is considered essential for providing patient care. Emphasis is placed on disease prevention, health promotion, and skills focused on caring for patients. The test is given over one day and can consist of varying numbers of questions and blocks, although the maximum amount of potential questions during the exam is 355 questions. The minimum passing score is 203 for Step 2 CK. Step 2 CK is usually taken at the end of the third or fourth year and is required by some schools prior to entering residency. Step 2 CK can, however, be taken at any time after passing USMLE® Step 1 providing eligibility requirements are met. Many students choose to take the USMLE® Step 2 CK at the beginning of the third year if they believe they can achieve a high score which would make them more competitive for residency. For those who do this, and score below average, this approach can backfire as well.

USMLE® Step 2 Clinical Skills (CS) is utilized to demonstrate the ability to provide patient care under supervision utilizing medical knowledge and the clinical sciences. Basic patient-focused care is stressed with the goal of being able to provide effective and safe care. Standardized patients are used as test subjects so that physical examinations and information gathering can be assessed. This test is currently graded on a pass/fail basis.

USMLE® Step 3 concentrates on general medical practice and the clinical sciences with the goal of demonstrating that a student can safely provide unsupervised medical care. The ambulatory care setting is stressed during this step with the overarching goal to reflect general clinical situations, although inpatient vignettes are used as well. The focus is on managing therapies and on the evaluation of patient problems. Multiple choice questions and case simulations are utilized based on patient vignettes. This step is usually taken during the first year of residency but can be taken at any time during residency depending on the rules based on the state where the student has their training license. Individual states within the U.S. may have varying rules on when Step 3 can be taken depending on the citizenship and country where the medical education was obtained as well. Passing of Step 1, Step 2 CK, and Step 2 CS are prerequisites in order to take this test. Step 3 is generally considered the least difficult of the three steps and is taken over two days. Day one consists of 336 multiple choice questions divided into seven blocks and day two consists of 144 multiple choice questions divided over four blocks. Included in the second day is testing based upon case simulations which utilize a Primum® Tutorial which involves a 15 minute instructional period followed by testing based directly on twelve patient case presentations. The minimum passing score for Step 3 is 190.

Many schools in Central and South America will advertise their pass rate for first time test takers on the USMLE®. This can be a very important number and an indicator of the effectiveness of the school. A passing rate of at least 90% or greater is desirable. As mentioned earlier, many schools utilize internal testing where passing is required before a student can be "released" to take the actual USMLE® test; this is used to reflect a higher official passing rate than would be the case if all students were allowed to take the test. The USMLE® pass rate is an important issue and is a valid question that one should ask of the school during the interview process. Each school will prepare their students for the USMLE® and some schools have designed their entire curricula toward teaching directly for these exams.

ECFMG®

The Educational Commission for Foreign Medical Graduates (ECFMG®) was founded in 1956. This program is designed to certify the abilities and preparedness of graduates of medical schools located outside of the United States and is required in order to enter any residency or fellowship program in the United States. The Accreditation Council for Graduate Medical Education (ACGME) must accredit these residency and fellowship programs, but these are the same residencies and fellowships that United States medical graduates enter. An international medical graduate must also hold ECFMG® certification prior to sitting for Step 3 of the USMLE® and many states require this certification to obtain licensure to practice medicine in that state.

The ECFMG® certification process involves submission of an application which contains information on several different areas. An applicant must have graduated from a school listed in the International Medical Education Directory (IMED), have completed four academic credit years of medical education, and have taken and passed USMLE® Step 1, Step 2 CK and Step 2 CS. Time limits are in place as well regarding the length of time needed to pass each of these steps. ECFMG® applicants must also submit verified copies of transcripts and diplomas. The ECFMG® required a Clinical Skills Assessment which was initially added in 1998, but this requirement is now met by the USMLE® Step 2 CS.

The State Board of Medical Examiners grants the official license to practice medicine in each specific state. The policies of each State Board vary; therefore, each prospective student should contact the specific state in which they desire to practice medicine in for specific requirements. Licensure requirements will generally be the same as they are for United States graduates except for the need for international graduates to have ECFMG®, and at times, AMRCB® certification. The medical school attended must also be approved by the state and listed by the WHO. New York and California have the strictest policies regarding licensure for international graduates.

The following tables display information on USMLE® performance for U.S and Canadian, and non-U.S. and Canadian test takers. Information for osteopathic trainees are included only if they have taken the USMLE®. Osteopathic physicians typically take the COMLEX® Steps 1, 2, and 3 and are not required to take the USMLE®. Many osteopathic students chose to take the USMLE®, however, in order to be more competitive for allopathic residencies and so that they can be compared directly with allopathic students who take only the USMLE® test series. It is noted that, in general, U.S. and Canadian medical school students score higher on USMLE® Step 1 on the initial attempt and when repeating the test than do non-U.S and Canadian students. This general trend holds true for USMLE® Step 2 CK, USMLE® Step 2 CS, and USMLE® Step 3. All subcomponent scores of the USMLE® Step 2 CS also note higher passing rates for U.S. and Canadian medical school students.

TABLE 2-A: Non-U.S. and Canadian School USMLE® Step 1 Performance

Non - U.S. and Canadian Schools	2012		2013	
	Number Tested	Percent Passing	Number Tested	Percent Passing
1st Attempt	14,201	76%	14,649	79%
Repeaters	4,261	40%	3,772	44%
Total	18,462	68%	18,421	72%

Source: Federation of State Medical Boards (FSMB) and National Board of Medical Examiners (NBME)

Table 2-B: U.S. and Canadian School USMLE® Step 1 Performance

U.S. and Canadian Schools	2012		2013	
	Number Tested	Percent Passing	Number Tested	Percent Passing
MD Degree	19,856	94%	20,023	95%
1st Attempt	18,723	96%	19,108	97%
Repeaters	1,133	68%	915	72%
DO Degree	2,564	91%	2,726	94%
1st Attempt	2,496	92%	2,680	94%
Repeaters	68	68%	46	74%
Total	22,420	94%	22,749	95%

Source: Federation of State Medical Boards (FSMB) and National Board of Medical Examiners (NBME)

TABLE 2-C: U.S. and Canadian School USMLE® Step 2 CK Performance

U.S. and Canadian Schools	2011-2012		2012-2013	
	Number Tested	Percent Passing	Number Tested	Percent Passing
MD Degree	18,929	97%	19,155	97%
1st Attempt	18,454	98%	18,658	98%
Repeaters	475	72%	497	74%
DO Degree	1,456	96%	1,634	96%
1st Attempt	1,439	97%	1,615	96%
Repeaters	17	53%	19	84%
Total	20,385	97%	20,789	97%

Source: Federation of State Medical Boards (FSMB) and National Board of Medical Examiners (NBME)

TABLE 2-D: Non-U.S. and Canadian School USMLE® Step 2 CK Performance

Non - U.S. and Canadian Schools	2011-2012		2012-2013	
	Number Tested	Percent Passing	Number Tested	Percent Passing
1st Attempt	11,908	85%	12,203	84%
Repeaters	2,191	54%	1,948	50%
Total	14,099	80%	14,151	80%

Source: Federation of State Medical Boards (FSMB) and National Board of Medical Examiners (NBME)

TABLE 2-E: Non-U.S. and Canadian School USMLE® Step 2 CS Performance

Non - U.S. and Canadian Schools	2011-2012		2012-2013	
	Number Tested	Percent Passing	Number Tested	Percent Passing
1st Attempt	11,515	80%	12,083	76%
Repeaters	2,265	65%	2,393	59%
Total	13,780	77%	14,476	73%

Source: Federation of State Medical Boards (FSMB) and National Board of Medical Examiners)

TABLE 2-F: U.S. and Canadian School USMLE® Step 2 CS Performance

U.S. and Canadian Schools	2011-2012		2012-2013	
	Number Tested	Percent Passing	Number Tested	Percent Passing
MD Degree	17,118	97%	20,201	97%
1st Attempt	16,662	97%	19,757	98%
Repeaters	456	92%	444	80%
DO Degree	46	87%	66	89%
1st Attempt	45	87%	63	89%
Repeaters	1	NA	3	NA
Total	17,164	97%	20,267	97%

Source: Federation of State Medical Boards (FSMB) and National Board of Medical Examiners (NBME)

TABLE 2-G: USMLE® Step 2 CS Subcomponent Passing Rates

Subcomponents: Integrated Clinical Encounter (ICE), Communication and Interpersonal Skills (CIS), Spoken English Proficiency (SEP)

	2011-2012			2012-2013		
	ICE	CIS	SEP	ICE	CIS	SEP
All US/Canadian Schools	98%	99%	>99%	98%	99%	>99%
All Non-US/Canadian Schools	86%	89%	97%	81%	92%	97%

Source: Federation of State Medical Boards (FSMB) and National Board of Medical Examiners (NBME)

TABLE 2-H: U.S. and Canadian School USMLE® Step 3 Performance

U.S. and Canadian Schools	2012		2013	
	Number Tested	Percent Passing	Number Tested	Percent Passing
MD Degree	19,056	95%	19,886	96%
1st Attempt	18,172	96%	19,086	97%
Repeaters	884	69%	800	78%
DO Degree	16	100%	25	92%
1st Attempt	16	100%	23	96%
Repeaters	0	N/A	2	NA
Total	19,072	95%	19,911	96%

Source: Federation of State Medical Boards (FSMB) and National Board of Medical Examiners (NBME)

TABLE 2-I: Non-U.S. and Canadian School USMLE® Step 3 Performance

Non - U.S. and Canadian Schools	2012		2013	
	Number Tested	Percent Passing	Number Tested	Percent Passing
1st Attempt	8,500	83%	8,781	87%
Repeaters	2,006	56%	1,978	64%
Total	10,506	78%	10,759	83%

Source: Federation of State Medical Boards (FSMB) and National Board of Medical Examiners (NBME)

TABLE 2-J: International Medical Student 2012 USMLE® Step 1 Performance

	Step 1	Step 2 CK	Step 2 CS
U.S. Citizen First Attempt	3983	3151	3343
U.S. Citizen Repeaters	1676	854	488
International Citizen First Attempt	10,184	8761	8175
International Citizen Repeaters	2587	1337	1781

Source: Federation of State Medical Boards (FSMB) and National Board of Medical Examiners

TABLE 2-K: Overall 2011-2012 USMLE® Step 1 and Step 2 Performance

	U.S. and Canadian Students	International Medical Students
Step 1 First Attempt	96%	76%
Step 1 Repeaters	68%	40%
Step 2 CK First Attempt	98%	85%
Step 2 CK Repeaters	71%	54%
Step 2 CS First Attempt	97%	80%
Step 2 CS Repeaters	92%	65%

Source: Federation of State Medical Boards (FSMB) and National Board of Medical Examiners (NBME)

AMRCB®

The American Medical Residency Certification Board (AMRCB®) was created to formalize the process of recognizing international excellence in medical education. The AMRCB® provides certification for international medical schools and for international medical students and graduates. The AMRCB® operates under the principle that many graduates of international medical institutions desire to practice medicine in a location other than the country where they attended medical school. The scope of the AMRCB® is to recognize the value of international medical training programs and their graduates within the United States.

The initial concept for the AMRCB® was conceived in the 1990's. A consortium was called of practicing physicians from the United States and the international community to establish and define the policies and procedures that would be necessary in order to appropriately understand the medical training that occurs across the globe. Through this effort, the official certification process for medical institutions and for medical students who desire to enter programs within the United States was begun in 2013.

For international medical students, it is not mandated that all have AMRCB® certification prior to entering a medical training program within the United States at this time. It is, however, being adopted by multiple agencies and organizations at this time. The majority of students take the course during their third and fourth year clinical rotations as they are applying to U.S. residency positions. Many others choose to take the course early on during their educational journey. The course is not focused on specific medical topics, but on professionalism, presentation skills, the ability to apply information and knowledge, attention to detail, communication skills, motivation, organization, and the ability to relate to people. The AMRCB® emphasizes the concept that professional skills are the foundation of success not only in the field of medicine, but in every successful organization. AMRCB® certification will help international graduates who seek to be distinguished from the large pool of yearly applicants for internship and residency positions, and for those who want to achieve a mark of excellence.

AMRCB® student certification can be achieved at any time during the medical education process. It may be taken before, during, or after the USMLE® and

ECFMG® testing and requirements. The AMRCB® differs from the ECFMG® as the AMRCB® provides focused qualitative assessment and training that evaluates multiple different professional skills necessary for the practice of medicine in the U.S. All applicants who undergo the certification process will not receive it, although the vast majorities who attend and complete the conference do receive certification. Conference attendees receive a qualitative assessment and are ranked among those who have completed the course. A transcript of the educational scores and assessments are available to the student and are sent, upon request, to individual U.S., Canadian, and international medical residencies and other organizations as well.

TABLE 2-L: AMRCB® 2013-2014 Certification Pass Rates

	U.S. and Canadian Students	International Medical Students
AMRCB First Attempt	95%	91%
AMRCB Repeaters	98%	88%

Source: AMRCB® 2014 Data Report

TRANSFERRING TO THE UNITED STATES

Many students who matriculate into Central and South America medical schools do so with the desire to transfer back to a United States medical school. This is possible but not probable. The competition for the few open spots in the United States is fierce. Most schools will have, at most, one or two open spots, and applicants for these spots often have to be residents of the state where the school is located. If a spot becomes open, the school wants to fill it, but they will do so with the most qualified candidate they can find. Transfer students will also usually have to take a series of competency tests on the basic sciences to prove that they have the ability to continue their education at that school. These tests are often held over the summer resulting in a loss of the vacation time that others will enjoy. It is also not uncommon for transfer students to be required to repeat the entire second year of the basic sciences at the school that has allowed the transfer. Step 1 USMLE® scores and AMRCB® certification will also be necessary for a transfer and the results of these tests should be exemplary. Some United States institutions may require that coursework taken at international institutions be evaluated for equivalence at United States institutions.

Course work evaluation companies have been established in order to identify the U.S. equivalency of education completed internationally. Students with academic transcripts from outside the U.S. and Canada must have their academic transcripts evaluated on a course-by-course basis by an evaluation service that is a National Association of Credential Evaluation Services (NACES) member (www.naces.org). These companies will determine if a student meets specific requirements by the educational institutions that they desire to transfer to. This process will involve the completion of many documents and the English translation of all non-English documents. The process seeks to identify the periods of study, verify diplomas and certificates, to determine U.S equivalency of semester credits, and the individual and overall grade point averages.

Table 2-M

Course Work Evaluation Companies

Josef Silny & Associates, Inc.
International Education Consultants

U.S. Mailing Address	Courier Address
Suite 241	P.O. Box 248233
1320 South Dixie Highway	Coral Gables, FL 33124
Coral Gables, FL 33146-2911	(305) 666-0233

Telephone: (305) 666-4133   e-mail: info@jsilny.org

Fax: (305) 666-0233   website: http://jsilney.com

World Education Services, Inc.
P. O. Box 745
Old Chelsea Station
New York, NY 10113-0745

Telephone: (212) 219-7335
Telephone: 800-937-3895   e-mail: mdobrow@wes.org
Fax: (212) 966-6393   website: http://www.wes.org

Intl. Education Research Foundation, Inc.
P.O. Box 66940
Los Angeles, CA 90066
(310) 390-6276

e-mail: contact via website
website: http:// ierf.org

Educational Credential Evaluators, Inc.
P.O. Box 514070
Milwaukee, WI 53203-3470
(414) 289-3400

Telephone: (414) 289-3412 ext. 110
Fax: (414) 289-3411

e-mail: lmartinez@ece.org
website: http://www.ece.org

American Council on Education (ACE)
One DuPont Circle NW
Washington DC, 20036-1193

Telephone: (202) 939-9300
Fax: (202) 833-4760

e-mail: web@ace.nche.edu
website: http://www.acenet.edu

American Association of Collegiate Registrar's and Admissions Officers (AACRAO)

One DuPont Circle, NW, Suite 520

Washington, DC 20036-1135

Telephone: (202) 296-3359

Fax: (202) 822-3940

http://www.aacrao.org

e-mail: oies@aacrao.org

website:

The low attrition rate in the United States is by design. Students have worked extremely hard to obtain medical school positions and will do everything to avoid losing their place. Medical schools in the U.S. also work very hard to prevent students from failing out due to the public and private money that is invested in the education of each student. Spots will, however, still become available. Many U.S. schools offer a remediation program for students having difficulty or for those who have failed classes. These students will often be allowed to repeat year one or year two and to continue their education. This results in openings for the clinical years while no students have actually left the program. The easiest schools to transfer into will be the schools who offer this opportunity for their students. This is still a difficult process and one that only a few students navigate successfully. Do not go to Central and South America thinking that you will definitely transfer back into the United States: this most likely will not happen.

PRACTICING IN THE UNITED STATES

One more thing that must be considered by applicants and graduates of medical schools located in the Caribbean region is whether or not the school that they attended is approved by the State or Province that they desire to eventually practice in. No single standard exists in the United States or Canada in regards to physician licensing regulations. Licensure is controlled by individual boards in all 13 provinces in Canada and all 50 states in the U.S. The regulations and requirements are frequently changed as well which can be challenging to prospective applicants. Terms such as "approved by California" or "recognized by New York" are often used. The educational quality of schools is determined by individual states and only this will allow for eventual licensure and practice upon graduation in specific areas.

Some states in the U.S. are considered to be leaders in this area. Approval from the Medical Board of California and the New York Education Department are very important. This recognition is often one of the first hurdles for Caribbean medical schools to overcome in order to provide clinical rotations and for graduates to obtain residencies in these states. In addition, approval by the National Committee of Foreign Medical Education (NCFMEA) and the Caribbean Accreditation Authority for Education in Medicine and Other Health Professions (CAAM-HP) are utilized by some states to determine eligibility.

Only a handful of Caribbean and Central and South American medical schools are approved by the Medical Board of California. In additional, several states directly follow the recommendation of California such as Colorado, Indiana, Kansas, and Oregon. California also maintains a "disapproved list" as well which can negatively affect schools for many years. School's generally take a decade to become approved by the state of California.

Table 2-N: U.S. State Licensure Approval References

State	Follow California Approved List	Reference California Disapproved List	Reference California Approved List	Follow Other
Alaska	Yes			
Alabama		Yes		
Colorado			Yes	CAAM-HP
Connecticut				WHO
Indiana		Yes	Yes	IMED/FAIMER, ECFMG
Louisiana				IMED/FAIMER WHO
Maine				IMED/FAIMER
Minnesota				IMED/FAIMER
New Jersey				IMED/FAIMER
New Mexico	Yes			
North Dakota		Yes		
Rhode Island				WHO
Tennessee			Yes	
Vermont		Yes		

Other states have approval lists as well which includes Florida, New Jersey, and Texas, although the lists in these states are not all encompassing. The individual laws pertaining to clinical rotations, residency eligibility, and eventual licensure eligibility vary in these as well as other states. Kansas and Idaho also require that an international school has been in operation for a minimum of 15 years.

A valuable reference for applicants is published by the American Medical Association entitled: *State Medical Licensure Requirements and Statistics 2014. ISBN#: 978-1-60359-897-2.*

Central and South American Medical Schools - Caribbean Region

Chapter 3
The Application Process

To attend a medical school in Central and South America applications must be made independently with each individual school. No centralized application service exists as it does in the United States. Because of this, no guidelines are in place which applies to all schools. Consequently, no secondary applications are usually needed because applications are filed directly through the schools. Application deadlines will vary, and applications can most often be submitted year-round.

Letters of recommendations will be required. Students are most often required to have two to five letters of recommendations forwarded to the individual schools. Several schools request a specific number of recommendations only, and a student should send only the number requested. Of the letters of recommendations, letters are often required from science faculty, advisors, and pre-medical committees if the student's school has one of these.

Do not assume that all material and items sent to the schools have been received. A student should, using care not to be overbearing, call and check that items have arrived at the schools and that their file is complete and the application is being processed. Countless students have been disqualified from applying after the application deadline has passed simply because a transcript or letter of recommendation was never sent, lost in the mail, or misplaced by the school.

Once the application is complete, each school will individually contact the students they are interested in to schedule an interview.

Older, non-traditional students are often apprehensive about applying to medical schools. This concern is unfounded, as non-traditional students are found in large numbers throughout United States, Caribbean, and Central and South America medical schools. Due to the different requirements of Caribbean and Central and South America schools, however, non-traditional students are usually found in larger numbers throughout these institutions. Central and South America medical schools seek students who are mature and who have had many life experiences.

MCAT®

The Medical College Admissions Test (MCAT®) is arguably the most difficult standardized test that any student will attempt in any discipline. The MCAT® has been offered for over 80 years and is now offered over 30 times each year at multiple locations in the U.S, Canada, and internationally, where it had previously been offered only twice a year. This author strongly recommends that applicants take the MCAT® in the spring of their junior year so that if they are dissatisfied with their test scores, they can retake it again later in the year. An applicant's knowledge of the sciences in general biology, general inorganic chemistry, organic chemistry, and general physics is tested. The overall content is tested with multiple choice questions and is divided over three scored, and one un-scored section. Overall reading comprehension and quantitative reasoning are also assessed. A student's writing abilities are still currently tested, although this is currently being revised and will no longer be included in the near future.

The MCAT® is required by all medical schools in Canada and the U.S. and is used and/or required by many international medical schools. The MCAT® is often used by other graduate and health professional programs as well and is currently taken by over 85,000 students each year. Successful completion of the MCAT® is currently identified a key to future success in medicine. The overarching goal is to assess a student's problem solving and critical thinking skills.

The MCAT® is currently undergoing major revisions currently planned to take place in 2015. The MCAT® is standardized and is offered in a multiple choice format so that all students can be evaluated using the same criteria. The Association of American Medical Colleges (AAMC) contracts with physicians, undergraduate university faculty, medical school faculty, and other experts to develop the test each year. The MCAT® underwent changes in 1991 so that the MCAT® of today is significantly different and includes more passages concerning the humanities and the social sciences than were previously available.

During each testing session, multiple versions of the MCAT® are given. Many of the passages students will receive will be the same, but several will be completely different. Although there will be content differences from test to test, the principles being tested are the same. No notes, calculators, or outside sources are permitted to be used during the testing. Total time to take the test, including breaks, is just over five hours.

The MCAT® currently consists of four sections, which are the Physical Sciences, Biological Sciences, Verbal Reasoning, and either the current Writing Sample or the new Trial Section depending on when the test is taken. All students who are preparing to apply to a health professions school are eligible to take the MCAT® which includes: Allopathic, Podiatric, Osteopathic, and Veterinary medicine. Students will be asked to accept a statement that verifies they are taking the exam only for the purpose of applying to a health professions school. Students who are currently enrolled in a medical school or those not planning on applying to a health profession school will require special permission to take the test. The requirements to sit for the test are the same for U.S., Canadian, and international medical students.

Prospective MCAT® applicants will be required to have an AAMC ID, user name, and password in order to register for the examination. The current cost of the exam is dependent upon when a student registers and if they are eligible for fee assistance. Fee assistance is designed for applicants who would not be able to take the exam or apply to medical school without this assistance. Those eligible for fee assistance also get a free copy of the Official Guide to the MCAT® Exam, and access to The Official MCAT® Self-Assessment Package.

For those applying without fee assistance greater than one month before the exam, the cost is $275 USD with a $65 USD fee to reschedule. For students applying two to three weeks prior the exam without fee assistance, the cost is $275 USD and a $125 USD fee to reschedule. Applicants who apply one to two weeks prior to the exam without fee assistance are charged $325 USD and are not eligible to reschedule at a lower fee. For those who are eligible for fee assistance and apply greater than one month before the exam, the cost is $100 USD with a $25 USD fee to reschedule. For students applying two to three weeks prior the exam with fee assistance, the cost is $100 USD and a $45 USD fee to reschedule. Applicants who apply one to two weeks prior to the exam with fee assistance are charged $150 USD and are not eligible to reschedule at a lower fee.

The exam will be given in order starting with the Physical Sciences, followed by Verbal Reasoning, Biological Sciences, and finally the current writing sample or the new Trial Section. The grading design is being changed to reflect a range of 1 to 15 for each section which will then be converted overall to a score ranging from 1 to 15 as well. The lowest score is reflected with a one, and the highest score is a fifteen.

The Physical Sciences section is constructed so that information learned in the first year courses of general physics and general inorganic chemistry is tested. The physics tested is not calculus based. This section of the MCAT® is given in 70 minutes, consists of 52 questions, and covers passage-based questions and non-passage-based questions. The scientific information is presented in passages, charts, graphs, and tables. Scientific problem solving is emphasized as is the interpretation of data. The questions given are generally 50% physics related and 50% chemistry related, but this can vary with each individual test and over individual years. Some MCAT® scores have been distributed by as much as 70/30 on these topics.

The Verbal Reasoning section is constructed so that the critical thinking, comprehension, and reasoning abilities of the applicant are tested. This section of the MCAT® is given over 60 minutes and consists of 40 questions. All of the questions in this section are passage-based. The passages can contain information about virtually any subject matter to include the social sciences and the humanities, as well as the physical sciences. Knowledge of specific subjects is not a prerequisite because all of the answers can be found in, or gleaned from, the passages.

The Biological Sciences section is presented in much the same manner as the Physical Sciences. This section of the test is constructed so that information learned in the first year courses of general biology and organic chemistry is tested. This section is also given over a 70 minute period, consists of 52 questions, and covers passage-based and non-passage-based questions. This information is presented with passages, charts, graphs, and tables. The subject matter tested is usually distributed 50/50 on biology and organic chemistry questions, but this is also variable.

The Trial Section is currently an un-scored section and will consist of 32 questions and will be given over 45 minutes. This section is voluntary and those who choose to take it currently will receive compensation. It is the last section tested during the exam. The Trial Section will consist of questions in either biochemistry, biology, chemistry, and physics; or in biology, psychology, and sociology. Questions in the Trial Section are generated based on responses given earlier in the exam.

The Writing Sample section will no longer be included as part of the MCAT® in 2015. In place of the Writing Sample, the current voluntary un-scored Trial Section is being used which initially began in 2013. The Writing Sample was constructed so that the students would complete two separate handwritten essays. Both essays had to be completed within 60 minutes, with each essay being completed individually within 30 minutes. This process was designed so that students could display their proficiency in writing and in their analytical skills. The essay topics did not require any prerequisite knowledge of subject matter and related to virtually any subject. Subjects that were sensitive, emotional, or offensive were not included in the essay topics.

Students will have the option on test day to release their scores to specific schools or to have their scores voided. The scores for the Biological, Physical, and Verbal sections are given on a range of 1 to 15. The scores of all students who take the MCAT® are processed. The scores are distributed basically along a parabolic curve so that only a few of the students who score poorly will receive 1's, and only a few of those who have perfect scores will receive 15's. The Writing Sample was scored on a range from "J" through "T". Each individual essay was graded on a range from 1-6 with a maximum of 12 total points available. A "J" resulted from receiving 1 point, a "K" from receiving 2 points, and so on. The highest score, a "T", was achieved by receiving 11 or 12 points. Students are able to retake the exam if they are not satisfied with the scores that they achieve, and many students choose to take a preparatory course in order to adequately prepare for the test.

Students often wonder what scores are needed to gain acceptance into medical school. This is often difficult to determine as admissions criteria vary from year to year and for each individual medical school. The MCAT® scores are only a part of the total application, but they are most often a large part. Admissions committees will use these scores to determine which applicants will succeed in not only their university's curriculum, but prospectively on the USMLE® licensing exams as well. Each school will have their own methodology of evaluating MCAT® scores. Some schools will consider the highest set of scores, some will use the highest score in each testing area, some will average all the scores, and some will weigh all scores equally. The MCAT® is just one part of the overall application one uses to apply to medical school. Other factors include the overall and science grade point averages (GPA's); letters of recommendation; the medical school interview; the difficulty and breadth of the undergraduate education; extracurricular activities; overall attitude and diversity; personal statements; and work, research, and volunteer related medical activities. Scores on the Verbal and the Science sections will usually need to be in the range of 7-10 to gain acceptance. Writing Sample scores usually need to be in the range of an "O" to gain acceptance. This is not, however, always the case. Students with overall scores in the low 20's and with writing scores of "L's" and "M's" are accepted every year. Many schools have MCAT® cutoff scores that a student must meet in order to apply. Cutoff scores are usually in the mid-20's and writing cutoff scores are often set at an "M" or an "O".

The bottom line is that although a low MCAT® score will not prevent a solid applicant from gaining acceptance into medical school, a very high MCAT® score can nearly cement a place for the well-rounded student. The MCAT® scores of applicants in Central and South America have historically been lower than for the students accepted in the United States. It is still of paramount importance for prospective applicants to study for and to take the MCAT® very seriously. Higher scores can result in higher degrees of success. It is also important to understand that not all Central and South America medical schools require the MCAT® be taken to gain acceptance into medical school. Many more schools require it now than did a decade ago, but it is still possible to be accepted into medical school in Central and South America without ever having taken the MCAT®.

PERSONAL STATEMENT

The personal statement that is presented on the application is very important. This statement is the opportunity for the prospective student to state their reasons for seeking a degree in medicine, as well as any other reasons that the student may feel are important to include. This will be the primary opportunity for medical schools to evaluate the applicant's writing proficiency, intelligence, motivation, thoroughness, and overall reasons for pursuing medicine. Students should take their time creating this statement and spend as much time on this as on any other part of the application process. The personal statement should be read, proofread, perfected, and reread. The statement should be read by as many persons as possible such as family members, friends, professors, and college staff if possible. Any grammatical mistakes or miswording will reflect extremely poorly on the applicant. Medical schools are not looking for students who are sloppy, careless, or do not take the proper time to effectively complete a written document.

The personal statement should reflect the reasons the student is pursuing medicine. Countless students have produced eloquent displays of grammatical perfection that stated nothing about why they wanted to become a physician. Medical schools want to know why you want to be a physician; do not leave this out. Students often choose to tell a story, use quotations, and to weave intricate personal descriptions into their personal statements. This is fine. A poignant description of a personal tragedy, the death of a loved one, or the humanistic issues witnessed during volunteer or work experiences may give the applicant depth. Uniqueness and interesting statements will also catch the eyes of the admissions board and may weigh in the student's favor. The student should be sure that the statement is cohesive, complete, and clearly describes the applicant. The difference in the personal statements of accepted medical students is extensive, but the common thread throughout is clarity and well-crafted writing.

APPLICANT CLASSIFICATION

Applicants to Central and South America medical schools will be classified as applicants from the North American system of education, the British system of education, or from all other systems of education. This classification will determine what specific requirements must be met in order to qualify for admission.

Applicants from the North American system of education are considered applicants from the United States and Canada. Course work will be required from an accredited college or university including at least 90 semester hours or 135 quarter hours. Preference is usually given to those who will have a baccalaureate degree upon matriculation. Although requirements for each school will vary, students should expect to have completed one full year of general biology, general chemistry, general physics, and organic chemistry. Courses in English, mathematics, and humanities are also often required.

Applicants from the British system of education must possess a strong science background. Applicants with passes at the advanced level of the General Certificate of Education will be considered. Applicants are assessed individually and students should have excellent passes in biology, chemistry, math, and physics.

All other applicants will include those from any country other than the United States, Canada, and Great Britain. Applicants from countries with similar educational standards as are present in the United States, and those from countries with variations from these U.S. standards, will be evaluated individually by the admissions committees. Each applicant should meet the educational requirements for admission to medical school in their home country. All course work and diplomas should be translated into English. Any applicant whose native language is not English will usually be required to take and pass the Test of English as a Foreign Language (TOEFL®) test or the International English Language Testing System (IELTS™). Acceptable pass ranges may vary by institution, but in general, acceptable minimum scores on the TOEFL® are 600 (paper-based), 250 (computer-based), or 100 (internet-based). For the IELTS™ the general minimum passing score is 7.0 overall.

Many Caribbean and Central and South American medical schools offer premedical programs as well that allows students to complete the required prerequisite coursework necessary to gain acceptance into medical school. Most of these programs will guarantee acceptance to the medical school at that institution if certain grades are achieved and the program is satisfactorily completed.

Chapter 4

The Interview

The interview process can be a major hurdle to overcome and will be the primary opportunity for individual students to demonstrate their value. Interviews with Central and South America medical schools are conducted via telephone, through regional interviews, and in some cases in person. Although one interview is generally all that is required for most applicants, it may be necessary to have an interview by telephone as well as one in person. Regional interviews can be beneficial and are held in various regions throughout the United States and Canada, usually in major cities such as New York, Chicago, Miami, and Los Angeles. Regional interviews can significantly reduce the time and financial strains for candidates. Do not be afraid to ask to reschedule interviews if doing so will save you time and money. Students will not benefit from flying to Guyana on Monday and then back to Belize on Thursday.

The medical schools would prefer applicants to visit the school personally and meet the students, but they understand that financial constraints can prevent this. The interview method will depend on each school and can also vary between students depending upon academic qualifications. Acceptance is almost always offered only after an interview has taken place. The policies and procedures for the interview process are usually provided for the applicants upon receipt of the initial application. The school's admission office can provide clarification of procedures if necessary.

Keep in mind that once the school grants an interview, that they have already made the decision that the applicant has the overall qualities that the school is looking for. The interview is often used to weed out unstable and immature applicants as well as to select the most impressive candidates. The goal is to sell yourself; applicants should therefore be prepared to make a good sales pitch. Medical schools in Central and South America understand that they are often competing for applicants with other schools. Most interviews will be relaxed and interviewers generally do not have the goal of pinning applicants down. Any direct contact with a prospective school should be conducted in professional attire. Do not make the mistake of ever under-dressing.

An applicant should expect to be asked questions concerning their reasons for pursuing medicine and their personal and academic histories. The interview is also an opportunity to ask questions of the school which may be very important in choosing which school to attend. Be prepared to ask questions as this can show motivation and preparation, both of which are desirable qualities.

Applicants should be familiar with, and observe all, application procedures of the school and submit all necessary documents in a timely manner. The medical schools should be kept informed of any change of address or telephone number. Applicants should promptly respond to invitations for an interview and promptly notify the school immediately if the interview needs to be cancelled or rescheduled.

BEFORE THE INTERVIEW

Be Prepared - Do not go into the interview without having practiced. Mock interviews and well thought out answers will be extremely beneficial. Also, students should be up-to-date on current events, as these questions are fair game. Newspapers and magazines will help applicants to prepare for these questions. It is particularly helpful to have researched information on the specific medical school, country, and region where the medical school is located.

Dress Professionally - The first impression that will be made will be the student's physical appearance. Men should dress in a dark suit with a tasteful tie and shined shoes. Suits should be black, blue, or gray and ties should not have any loud designs or colors. Women should wear dress coordinates or a suit, although a suit may not always be appropriate for all schools. Shoes should not have heels that are too high and make-up and jewelry should be tasteful. All students should have a leather binder with them for the information that they will receive.

Arrive Early - The absolute worst thing that a prospective student can do is to arrive late for an interview. All students should have several copies of their application and personal statement with them to hand out if requested and have reviewed these prior to arrival. Be familiar with the school catalog and with any programs of which the school is particularly proud. From the moment the student sets foot into the city they are interviewing in, they must treat everyone with the utmost respect. This applies particularly to the administrative staff and students of the school, because one never knows who the person they cut-off in the parking lot or were rude to at a restaurant may be. This may be one of the interviewers. One must also treat all support staff with respect, particularly the administrative and secretarial staff as they often will have direct input on prospective students, and are often vocal on the impressions they have of individual applicants.

DURING THE INTERVIEW

Be Self-Confident - Applicants should be self-confident but it no way pushy or overbearing. It is acceptable to be witty and charming, but not sarcastic. Often, the actual answer to a question is not nearly as important as the manner in which the question is handled. Poise and confidence will go a long way

Exhibit Control - Begin by acknowledging the interviewer by name, introduce yourself, and offer a handshake. Next, do not exhibit nervous movements. Fidgeting, talking too fast, shaking one's leg, or fondling a pen or brochure can be very irritating to the interviewer. Do not forget to maintain appropriate eye contact and to respond timely to comments or humor from the interviewer.

Answer Questions Intelligently - Think about what is going to be said before it is said. Stuttering or rambling while answering a question will cause the student to appear unintelligent. Do not answer questions with an attitude or like a know-it-all. Interviewers are not looking for students who know everything. If a student does not know an answer, they should say so. It will be much more beneficial to be honest than it will be to make something up and appear shallow and dishonest. If the interviewer wants to aggravate or antagonize the applicant, do not respond in the same manner. Stay calm and relaxed and understand that this is probably only a test to see how the applicant is going to react under stressful situations.

AFTER THE INTERVIEW

Remain Composed - After the interview, offer a handshake and say good-bye. Tell the interviewer that their time is appreciated. Be prepared to take a tour of the school and/or hospital. Composure during the tours and during lunch will be just as important as it is during the interview. The tour guides are usually medical school students and they may have input into the student's evaluation as well.

Send Thank-You Notes - Many students often skip this last step; do not be one of them. Sending thank-you notes gives the student one last chance to contact the school and to reiterate their interest and the desire to attend that school. Interviewers will appreciate this formality and it will help them to remember the student in a positive light. The best approach is to write the thank-you notes immediately after the interviews. Memories of the event, interactions, and specific content of individual discussions will fade over several hours to several days.

POSSIBLE INTERVIEW QUESTIONS

- What are your thoughts on the Accountable Care Act?
- How are you today? Did you have trouble locating us?
- Why do you want to be a doctor?
- Which field of medicine are you interested in?
- What kind of experiences do you have in the medical field?
- Where do you plan to practice medicine?
- What are your goals in medicine?
- Where do you see yourself in 5, 10, or 15 years?
- Why did you apply to our school?
- Would you go to our program if I gave you an acceptance letter right now?
- Why should we choose you over all of the other applicants?
- What will you bring to the class if you are accepted?
- What other programs have you applied to besides ours?
- Did anyone you know influence your career choice?
- Do you have family members who are physicians?
- Tell us your definition of a professional.
- If you were held up at gunpoint with a loved one, what would you do?
- What do you think of affirmative action?
- Give me an example of something you did that was wrong.
- Explain you research project.
- Would you get out of your car in a highway to help an accident victim?
- If an AIDS patient were bleeding profusely from an injury, what would you do?
- What do you think is the most difficult issue facing the medical community?
- What do you think of herbal or alternative medicine?
- What would you do if a family member decided to solely depend on alternative medicine for their treatment of a significant illness?
- How will you handle being taught something that you already know?
- Can you handle somebody throwing up on you?
- What are your thoughts on Medicare reform?
- How would you improve preventive healthcare settings?
- How would you improve access to healthcare in your country?
- Do you feel that the government should be involved with mandating insurance?
- How would you control the rising cost of healthcare?
- What interests do you have outside of medicine?

- Do you plan to continue your hobbies as you go through medical school?
- If you had one day to do anything, what would you do?
- What row in a classroom do you normally sit in and why?
- What was the last book that you read and would you recommend it?
- What was the last movie that you saw?
- What did you do in your last job?
- Which classes did you enjoy the most and why?
- How would your friends describe your personality?
- Do you have an autocratic personality?
- What are your strengths and weaknesses?
- What one thing would you change about yourself?
- Is there something about you that would make you difficult to get along with?
- What type of people do you get along with well?
- Describe the most exciting event of your life.
- What do you think will be the most difficult aspect of medical school?
- Why did you do so poorly in _____ (a particular class)?
- Do you think that your classes were enough to prepare you for our program?
- Imagine that you find a lamp that gives you three wishes. What would they be?
- You discover that one of your peers is abusing drugs. What would you do?
- What qualities would you look for in your doctor?
- What qualities would you look for in your patients?
- What would you do if a nurse refuses to carry out your orders?
- If you could be any animal, what would you be and why?
- If you could be any car, what would you be and why?
- Who do you admire the most in your life?
- If you could choose one figure in history to have dinner with, who would it be?
- Have you always put forth your best effort in every situation?
- Tell me about something that you know a lot about?
- You have just diagnosed a man with a sexually transmitted disease that he did not get from his wife. He says that he is not going to tell her. What would you do?
- If you find that the professor with whom you have done research has changed some of the data before publication, what would you do?
- During your clinical rotations, you treated a wealthy patient. He has decided to give you $100,000. What would you do with the money?
- What would you do if you saw a fellow medical student cheating on an exam?

- What are your thoughts on abortion?
- What are your thoughts on Euthanasia?
- How do you feel about fetal tissue research?
- How would you tell a patient that they have cancer?
- What would you do if your supervising doctor was under the influence of alcohol?
- A young teenager who is pregnant comes to you to discuss her options but says she has not told her parents about her pregnancy. How would you handle this?
- Do you think doctors are getting paid too much or too little?
- Do you think that decreasing the salaries of physicians can solve rising healthcare cost issues?
- What do you think about socialized medicine?
- What do you think of the doctor shortage/oversupply in different areas?
- What would you do if a doctor told you to give a medicine that you knew would harm the patient??
- Why do you think the number of applicants has been growing every year despite the problems we face in medicine?
- What would you do if you do not get into medical school this year?

QUESTIONS TO ASK

- What is the USMLE® pass rate on Step 1 and Step 2 for your school?
- Does your school offer, or require a USMLE® review course?
- What is your clinical placement rate inside of the United States?
- Is your school certified by the AMRCB®?
- With which hospitals does your school have an affiliation?
- Do students have to secure their own cadavers?
- How are students chosen for clinical rotations in certain locations?
- What percentage of your graduates obtain a residency in the United States?
- Are all of your facilities air-conditioned?
- What technology is available at your school?
- Are any scholarships and loans available at your school, and if so, which ones?
- How long will it take before I know if I am accepted?
- How frequent are power outages?
- If I am not accepted into the class of my choice, will I be given a choice of matriculating into a later class?
- If I am granted acceptance, does your school allow students to defer enrollment into a class at a later date?
- Do you have any school housing for singles and/or families?
- What loans are available for students at your institution?
- Are students required to live in on-campus housing for a required amount of time?
- What schools are available for my children?
- What clubs and support groups are available for my family?
- Is your institution a not-for-profit or a for-profit institution?
- Are textbooks, microscopes, etc. available on location from your school or do I have to ship them in from overseas?
- How many graduates have received the M.D. degree from your school?
- Has your school ever had to shut down due to financial or other reasons?
- Have you undergone, or will you soon be, changing the curriculum?
- How is the grading system designed?
- What year did the first medical school class start at your institution?
- Has your institution moved locations or islands in the past? If so, why?
- What percent of the graduating class secured residency spots upon graduation?

- How many students have transferred out of your program over the last 3 years?
- How many students have dropped out of your institution over the last 3 years? For what reasons?
- What selection criteria does your school use to select students?

Chapter 5

Residency

Obtaining a residency is the most important step in the journey of becoming a practicing physician. The Doctor of Medicine (M.D.) degree can be earned anywhere, but without a residency, the goal of practicing medicine in the United States will not be possible. The quest for a U.S. residency will be more difficult for physicians trained outside of the United States, but it is still possible. Currently, over 22.8% (175,000) physicians practicing in the United States attended medical school outside of the United States.

One of the primary reasons for the large number of internationally trained physicians who practice in the U.S. is the unmet need in the U.S. Over half of all internationally trained physicians in the world who practice in a host country work in the United States. Large inflows of physicians currently migrate to the U.S. from India, Pakistan, Eastern Europe, and the Philippines. While some countries such as France have less than 5% of their physician workforce made up of doctors who trained outside of their country, countries such as Ireland have over 33% of their physician workforce that come from other countries.

Each year, roughly 20,000 students graduate United States Allopathic and Osteopathic medical schools. Currently there are 26,392 U.S. residency positions available each year. This means that just fewer than 7,000 positions are available each year for graduates outside of the United States. Graduates are seeking these remaining 7,000 spots from all international medical schools and from Doctor of Osteopathy (D.O.) schools, regardless of their citizenship. On average, just over 20,000 independent applications are filed for the remaining 7,000 residency spots each year. Needless to say, competition is fierce, and any applicant desiring a residency position must have outstanding qualifications. Success is ultimately decided on personal abilities, references from the hospitals where the clinical clerkship rotations were completed, grades in medical school, USMLE® test scores, AMRCB® certification, and how well the student interviews for the residency on the phone and/or in person.

Virtually all U.S. residencies are obtained by utilizing the National Resident Matching Program (NRMP®). The first match began in 1952 with 10,400 positions available. Available positions had expanded to over 19,000 in 1973, and other than a brief decrease in positions after isolated internships were abolished in 1975, the positions have now risen to 26,392 positions in 2014. The trend of applications for these positions has risen sharply over the years as well from 6000 in 1952 to 40,335 in 2013. Applicants will need to officially apply as one of the following: U.S Allopathic seniors; previous U.S. allopathic graduates; graduates or students of Canadian medical schools; graduates or students of osteopathic medical school; graduates or students of Fifth Pathway Programs; U.S. citizen graduates or students of international medical schools; non-U.S. graduates and students of international medical schools; U.S. citizen and non-U.S citizen graduates and students of international medical schools; or as independent applicants. In addition, applicants can also apply as couples and for post graduate years (PGY) one and two.

The National Residency Matching Program (NRMP®) matches applicants seeking postgraduate residency positions in the United States with the institutions that offer these positions. Students rank their preferences confidentially as late as their senior year of medical school. The students are matched to training programs that rank the highest according to the selections that they have made and to those programs that have offered acceptances. Students and graduates of international medical schools may enroll in this program as an individual if they submit proof of having passed the ECFMG® required examinations by the submission date. International medical students can complete the ECFMG® application in the early Fall prior to the expected start date of residency programs in July. Candidates who intend to enter the United States as an exchange visitor must qualify and meet conditions under United States law and must be able to secure a visa.

Based on data from 2013, 96.4% of all positions were filled. Initially, 1041 positions were unmatched, and 939 of these positions were filled in the "scramble" now known as the SOAP® process. In 2013, 34,355 applications were filed for the available positions of which 26,392 were first year positions and 2779 were second year positions. U.S. allopathic seniors made up 17,487 of these applications which was nearly a 6% increase from 2012 and was a direct result of expanding medical school class sizes and the addition of several new allopathic and osteopathic medical schools. The largest increases in applications were from international medical school students who were U.S. citizens and graduates: these increased by 816 applications. A total of 5095 international medical students who were U.S. citizens applied through the match which is over 50% more than applied in 2009. Seniors from U.S. allopathic medical schools made up 93% of matches with nearly 80% matching to one of their top three choices. The match rate for U.S. osteopathic graduates and students was 75% and was the highest in three decades. Applications from non-U.S. international medical school graduates and students increased in 2013 as well to 7,568 from 6,828 in 2012. This was an increase in the match rate to over 47% from 40% the year before.

For the 2013 match, the vast majority of positions were in Family Medicine, Internal Medicine, Psychiatry, Anesthesiology, and Pediatrics. This group of specialties made up over 77% of the total number of match positions. International medical graduates and students who were U.S. citizens matched primarily into Internal Medicine (993 total positions) and Family Medicine (690 positions). In addition, international medical graduates and students who were U.S. citizens matched into the following disciplines: Psychiatry – 219, Pediatrics – 192, Surgery – 109, Anesthesiology – 100. For international medical graduates and students who were not U.S. citizens, matches were made in the following specialties: Internal medicine – 1199, Family Medicine – 385, Pediatrics – 290, Surgery – 214, Psychiatry – 186, Neurology – 174, and Pathology – 158.

Additional analysis of the most recent match data from 2013 notes that 93.7% of allopathic seniors from U.S. medical schools matched into a residency position. Reflecting the highest match rate since 2005, 53.1% of U.S. citizens who trained in international medical schools matched. The match rate for international medical school graduates and seniors who were not U.S. seniors rose dramatically to 47.6 percent. The top five specialties overall in the match were: Pediatrics (63.9%), Family Medicine (51.3%), Pathology (51.3%), Internal Medicine (49.5%), and Physical Medicine and Rehabilitation (49.5%).

Previously known as the "scramble," a new process called the Supplemental Offer and Acceptance Program (SOAP℠) is now in place. The SOAP® has been designed to streamline the process that is used to fill unmatched positions. Applicants are eligible for SOAP® when they have registered for the main match, become unmatched or partially matched, and are eligible to begin a residency on

July 1st of the match year. Those who have not submitted a rank order list are also eligible for this process. For applicants in 2013, 13,808 became eligible for the SOAP process. The majority of these applicants (greater than 40%) were international medical graduates that were not citizens of the United States, with U.S. citizen international medical graduates and students comprising 25%, and 15% respectively of U.S. Seniors. A total of 1,041 positions were left unmatched, with 939 of these becoming eligible for the SOAP process. Of these, 57.6% of positions (446 total) were for PGY-1. SOAP eligible positions included surgery, internal medicine, pediatrics, anesthesiology, family medicine, and diagnostic radiology. A total of 1,327 positions were offered to applicants of whom 878 were accepted resulting in a total match rate of 93.5%. The majority of the positions (67%) were filled with U.S. seniors.

Those who are not accepted into a regular residency via the match or the SOAP process can obtain some residencies from non-traditional sources. The military is an option but this is very limited for graduates outside of the United States. Only a small minority of the available military residencies are filled by individuals who were not enlisted during medical school. To find out about these military positions, students should contact the branch of service in which they are interested. Independent matches also exist and this can prove to be a viable option. This entails finding a private physician who is willing to establish a residency and work as the student's supervisor.

The advantage of attending a Central or South America medical school instead of other international medical schools is that many Central and South America schools are able to place their students in affiliated hospitals in the United States during clinical rotations in the third and fourth year. Residency programs often feel more comfortable with students that have been trained in United States hospitals and who are familiar with the technology and procedures in the United States. Students who have performed clinical rotations in the United States will benefit from making contacts and friendships with supervisors and other doctors. These relationships will allow the student to obtain letters of reference that can aid a student in obtaining a residency.

Central and South America schools also place many students in residencies throughout the Caribbean, Central and South American, the United Kingdom, and other areas across the globe according to differing criteria. Some students are placed by choice and availability, but the students placed in the United States are done so usually as a result of competition and grades. The overarching goal of most schools is to place students in the United States for clinical rotations. For an internationally trained physician, performance throughout the undergraduate and graduate education is very important when it comes to obtaining a residency. The USMLE® scores and AMRCB® certification are the most important as this shows competency and abilities in comparison to the students trained in the United States. An aspiring physician trained in the Central and South America with above average USMLE® scores and AMRCB® certification will be well on their way toward obtaining a residency.

United States residency programs are recognized by specialties and span from three to seven years depending upon the specialty. Some specialties require a one-year transitional year of residency prior to beginning the specialty years. A good online resource is the Fellowship and Residency Electronic Interactive Database Access System (FREIDA®). FREIDA® is a website that lists all ACGME approved residency programs. The "Green Book" also exists and is the official Graduate Medical Education Directory. A copy can be purchased through the American Medical Association. This book details all of the residency programs available in the United States and explains the licensure requirements that apply in each state. Certain hospitals, specialties, and geographic areas will be highly competitive while others will offer a much greater chance of acceptance.

Chapter 6
IMG Match Data

The data and material presented in this chapter is intended for review by international medical school graduates, international medical schools, and medical residencies located within the United States. Only data from International Medical School graduates are included. This data does NOT include U.S. medical school graduates other than in the initial Main Residency Match® graph (Table 1). Data are further divided by international medical school graduates who are U.S. citizens and those who are not U.S. citizens. It is further presented for those that did, and did not, match into a U.S. residency program in 2013. Information in the section is taken directly from the National Residency Match Program (NRMP®) and the American Medical Residency Certification Board (AMRCB®).

Data Summary

It is noted that international medical graduates who are successful in matching in their specialty of choice have several identifiable qualities. Statistically, those who are the most successful are as follows: speak English as a native language; have high USMLE® scores; have graduated from medical school and obtained AMRCB® and ECFMG® certification within one year of the match; are U.S. citizens; and rank multiple programs within their specialty of choice. This does not mean that students who do not meet these qualities will not obtain a residency position of their choice, but understanding what qualities are most often selected will allow applicants to make informed decisions and to identify areas of potential improvement.

For the 2013 match year, a total of 34,455 individuals participated in the residency match in the United States. In total, international medical graduates comprised 36.8% of these applicants. Of these, 7,568 were non-U.S. citizens while 5,095 were U.S. citizens.

Many international medical graduates will rank more than one specialty to increase the odds that they will match into a U.S. residency program. On average, those who matched ranked 1.4 specialties and those that did not match ranked 1.6 programs. The reason why those who did not match ranked, on average, more programs than those that did not is unclear. The specialty with the highest number of ranked specialties was anesthesiology and the specialty with the lowest number of ranks was Pathology.

On average, U.S. international medical graduates who matched in 2013 took the USMLE® Step 1 an average of 1.2 times compared with 1.7 times for those who did not match. For non-U.S. international medical graduates, those who matched took Step 1 of the USMLE® an average of 1.1 times and those that did not match took it an average of 1.2 times. The probability of matching into the specialty of choice was 0.52 for U.S. international medical graduates and 0.46 for international graduates who were non-U.S. citizens.

The mean number of Step 2 CK attempts was 1.1 attempts for U.S. international medical graduates who matched and 1.6 times for those who did not match. For non-U.S. international medical graduates taking Step 2 CK, the average number of attempts was 1.0 for those who matched and 1.2 for those that did not match. The probability of matching into the specialty of choice by USMLE® Step 2 CK scores was 0.54 for U.S. international medical graduates and 0.46 for non-U.S. international medical graduates. The mean number of USMLE® Step 2 CS attempts was 1.1 for U.S. international medical graduates who matched and 1.4 attempts for those who did not match. For non-U.S. international medical graduates, the mean number of attempts was 1.1 for those who matched and 1.3 for those who did not match.

Regarding ECFMG® certification, the mean number of months after certification was 8.0 for U.S international medical graduates who matched and 25.6 months for those who did not match. For non-U.S. international medical graduates, the mean number of months since ECFMG® certification was 16.0 for those who matched and 25.6 months for those who did not match.

The mean number of years after graduation was 1.7 years for U.S. international medical graduates who matched and 5.7 years for those who did not. For non-U.S. graduates, the average number of months since graduation was 4.7 years for those who matched and 7.5 years for those who did not match.

For those applicants whose native language is English, international medical graduates made up 76% of those who matched and 56% of those who did not match. For non-U.S. international medical graduates, 24% of those who matched spoke English as a native language and 18% of those who did not match spoke English as a native language.

Overall Main Residency Match

Table 6-A: 2013 Main Residency Match®

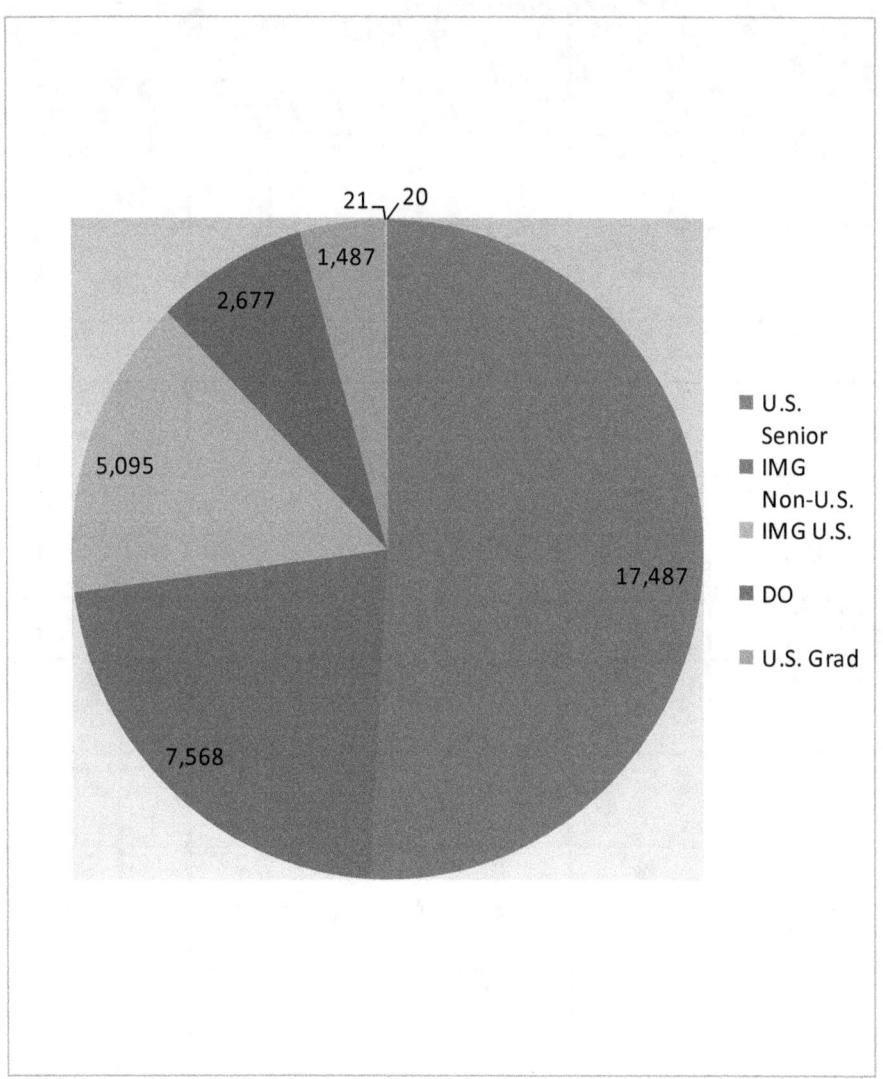

Source: NRMP® and ECFMG® Charting Outcomes in the Match for International Medical Graduates, 2014

Table 6-B: International Medical Graduate Applicants and Positions 2013 Main Match

Specialty	Total Positions	Total Applicants	Applicants Per Position	IMG U.S. Matched Yes / No		IMG Non-U.S. Matched Yes / No	
Internal Medicine	6612	9193	1.4	841	753	1690	1856
Family Medicine	3037	4096	1.3	53	137	31	53
Pediatrics	2699	3258	1.2	186	151	278	382
Emergency Medicine	1744	2219	1.3	53	137	31	53
Anesthesiology	1653	1846	1.1	95	65	78	85
Psychiatry	1362	1921	1.4	203	256	163	277
OB/GYN	1237	1613	1.3	78	99	62	120
General Surgery	1185	1872	1.6	119	123	158	150
Diagnostic Radiology	1143	1254	1.1	55	47	66	63
Neurology	692	844	1.2	59	44	148	149
Pathology	583	797	1.4	46	69	151	136
Physical Medicine and Rehabilitation	397	548	1.4	40	43	21	26

Source: NRMP® and ECFMG® Charting Outcomes in the Match for International Medical Graduates, 2014

Central and South American Medical Schools - Caribbean Region

Table 6-C: 2013 Match Applicant Mean Statistics

Statistic	IMG U.S.		IMG Non-U.S.	
	Matched	Un-Matched	Matched	Un-Matched
USMLE® Step 1 Score	217	204	227	213
USMLE® Step 1 Attempts	1.2	1.7	1.1	1.2
USMLE® Step 2 CK Score	224	209	233	218
USMLE® Step 2 CK Attempts	1.1	1.6	1.0	1.2
USMLE® Step 2 CS Attempts	1.1	1.4	1.1	1.3
Months Since ECFMG® Certification	8	26	16	26
Months Since AMRCB® Certification *	3.2	5.2	2.1	4.8
Years Since Graduation	1.7	5.7	4.7	7.5
Number of Ranks	7	3	6	3
Numbers of Specialties Ranked	1.4	1.6	1.3	1.5
Percent Native English Speakers	76	56	24	18

Sources: NRMP® and ECFMG® Charting Outcomes in the Match for International Medical Graduates, 2014; AMRCB® Certification Data Report – 2014
* AMRCB® certification began in 2013 which may affect comparison data

Table 6-D: USMLE® Step 1 Scores - All Matched U.S. Applicants

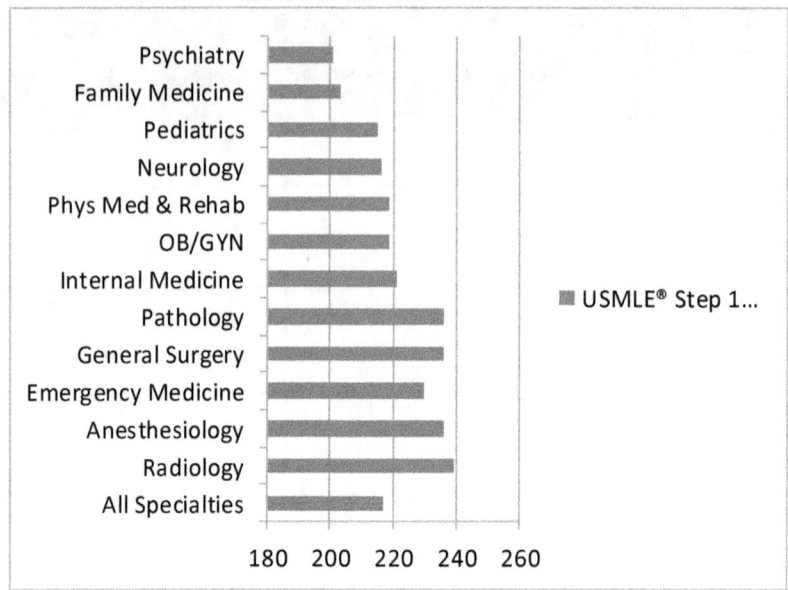

Source: NRMP® and ECFMG® Charting Outcomes in the Match for International Medical Graduates, 2014

Central and South American Medical Schools - Caribbean Region

Table 6-E: USMLE® Step 1 Scores - All Matched International Graduates

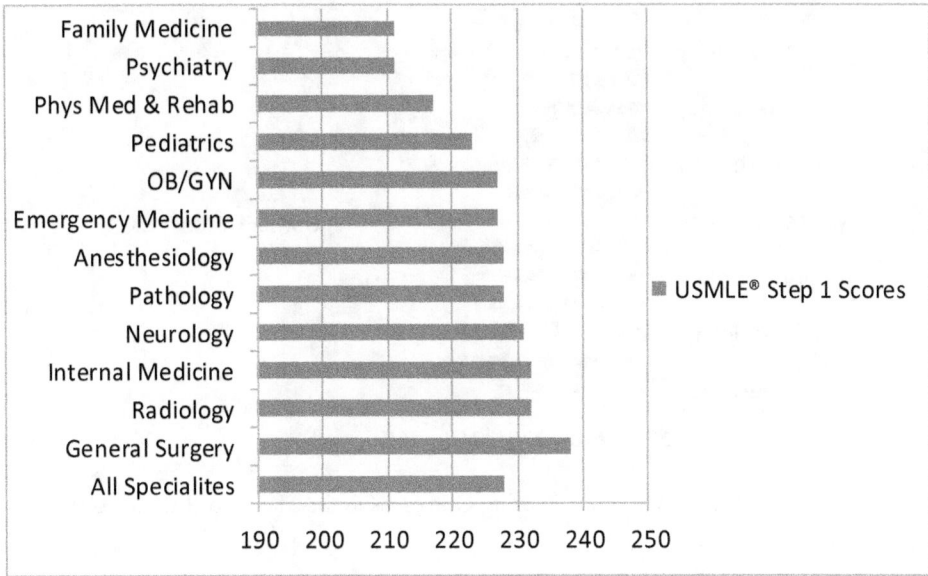

Source: NRMP® and ECFMG® Charting Outcomes in the Match for International Medical Graduates, 2014

Table 6-F: USMLE® Step 2 CK Scores - All Matched U.S. IMG's

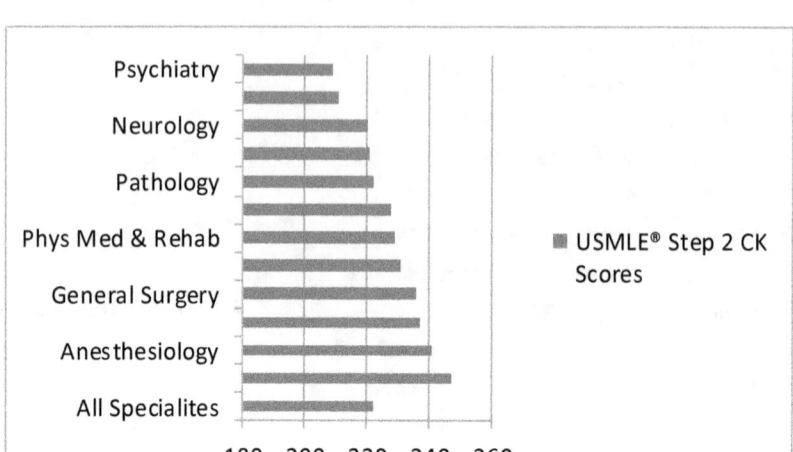

Source: NRMP® and ECFMG® Charting Outcomes in the Match for International Medical Graduates, 2014

Table 6-G: USMLE® Step 2 CK Scores - All Matched Non-U.S. IMG's

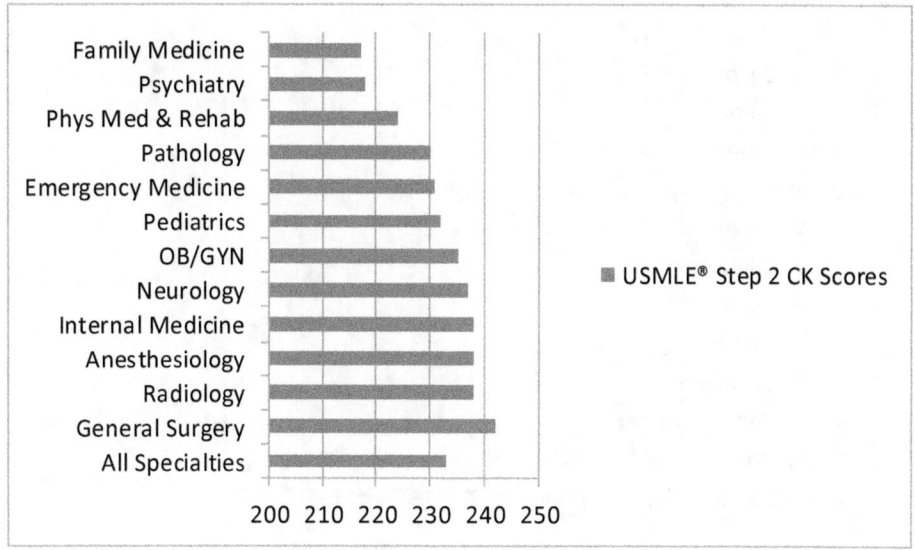

Source: NRMP® and ECFMG® Charting Outcomes in the Match for International Medical Graduates, 2014

Table 6-H: U.S. International Medical Graduates Citizenship at Birth 2013

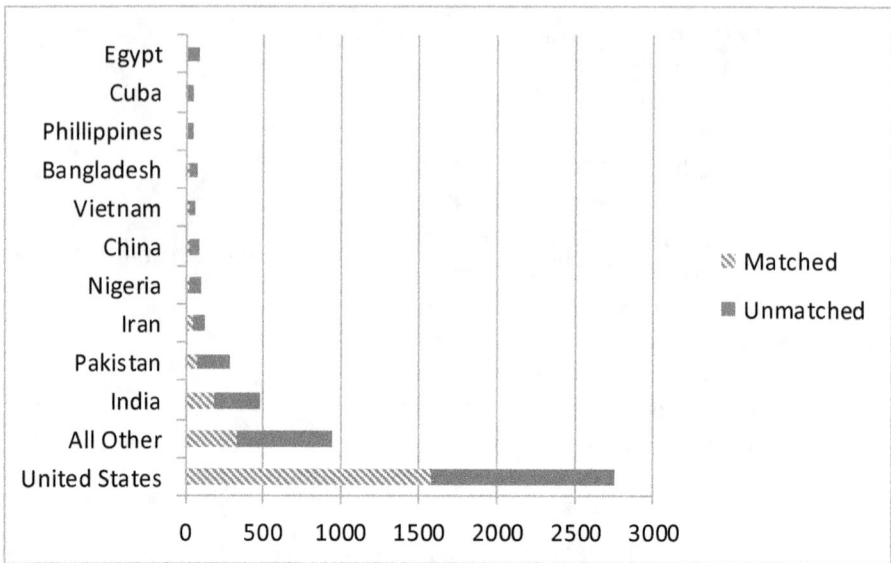

Source: NRMP® and ECFMG® Charting Outcomes in the Match for International Medical Graduates, 2014

Central and South American Medical Schools - Caribbean Region

Table 6-I: Non-U.S. International Medical Graduate Citizenship at Birth 2013

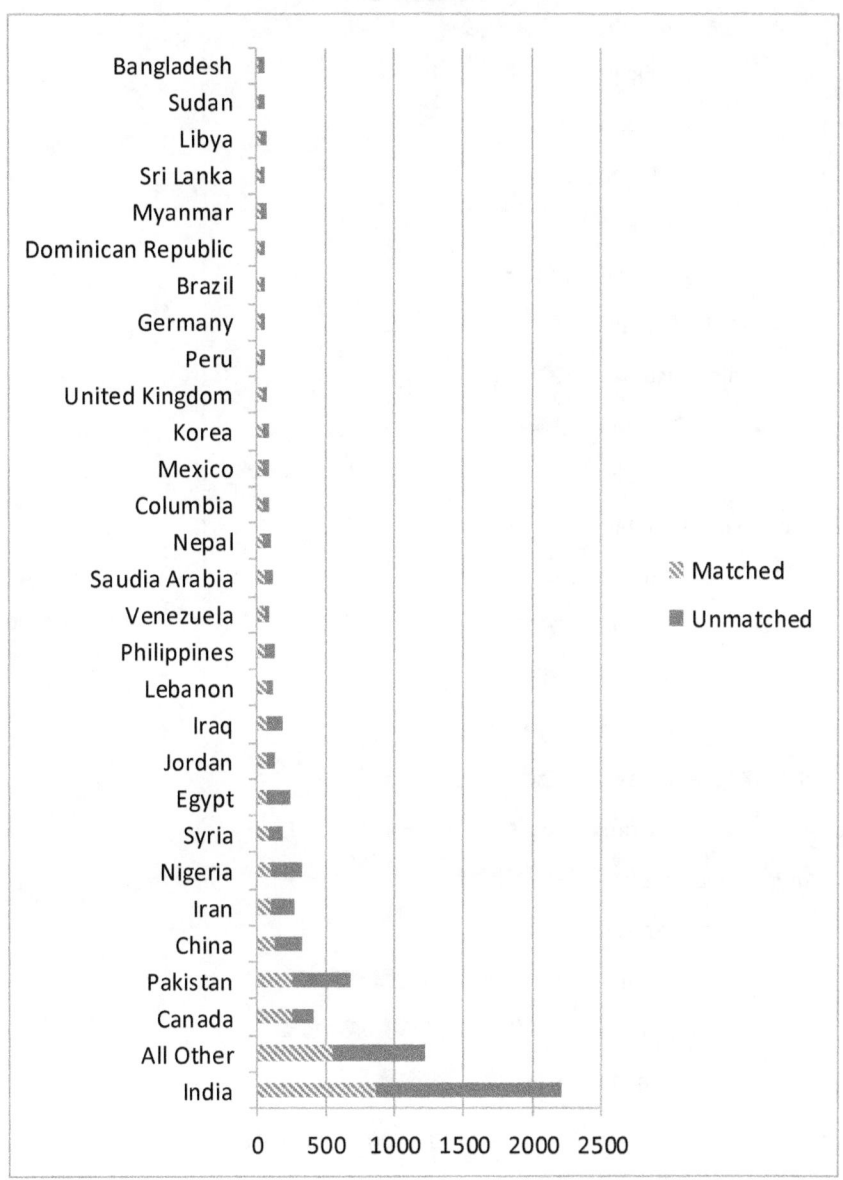

Source: NRMP® and ECFMG® Charting Outcomes in the Match for International Medical Graduates, 2014

Central and South American Medical Schools - Caribbean Region

Table 6-J: U.S. International Medical Graduates - Country of Medical School 2013

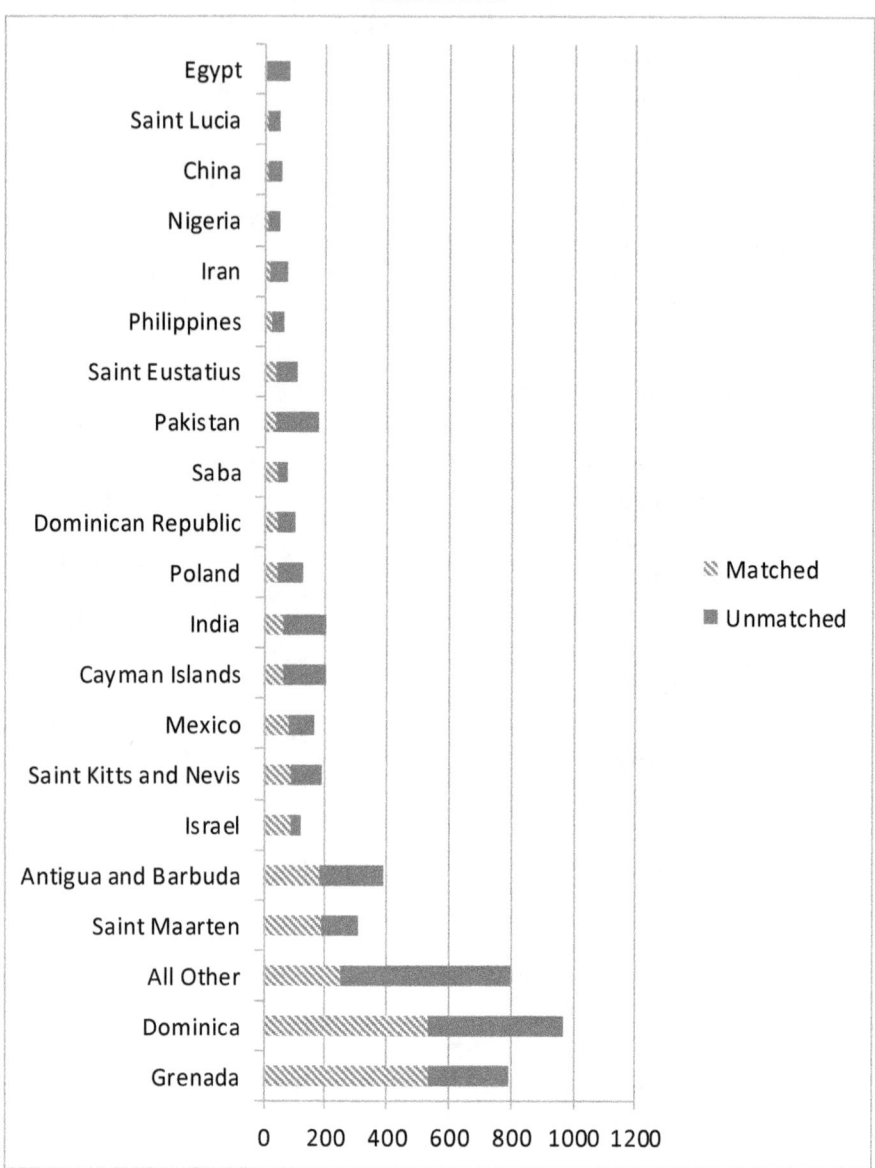

Source: NRMP® and ECFMG® Charting Outcomes in the Match for International Medical Graduates, 2014

Table 6-K: Non-U.S. International Medical Graduates - Country of Medical School 2013

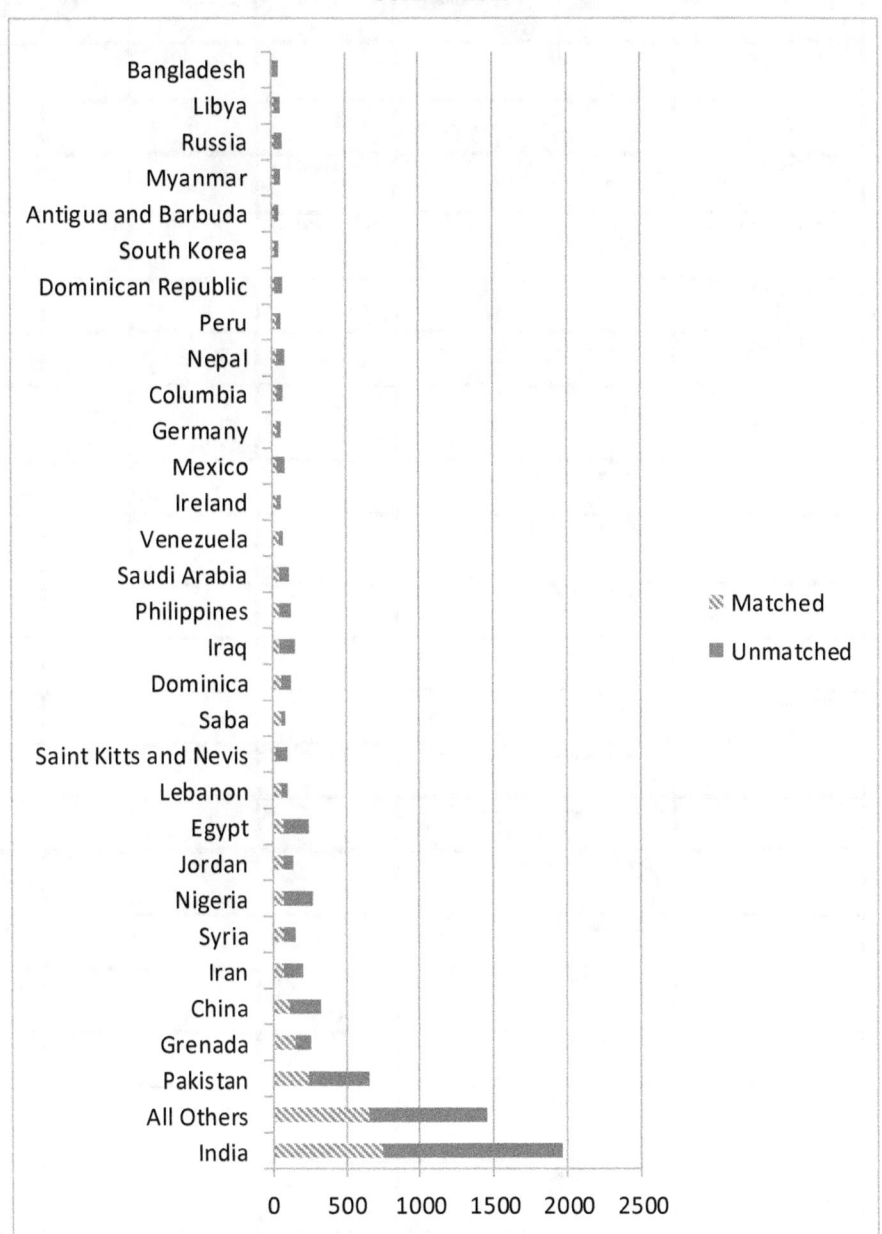

Source: NRMP® and ECFMG® Charting Outcomes in the Match for International Medical Graduates, 2014

Central and South American Medical Schools - Caribbean Region

Table 6-L: LENGTH OF UNITED STATES RESDENCIES

Year 1	Year 2	Year 3	Year 4	Year 5	Year 6	Year 7
Family Practice						
Emergency						
Pediatrics			Sub-specialties			
Internal Medicine			Sub-specialties			
OB/GYN						
Pathology						
General Surgery				Sub-specialties		
	Neuro-Surgery					
	Orthopedic Surgery					
	Otolaryngology					
	Urology					
Transitional Year						
	Dermatology					
	Neurology					
	Nuclear Medicine					
	Ophthalmology					
	Physical Medicine					
	Psychiatry					
	Radiology Diagnostic					
	Radiation Oncology					

AVERAGE U.S. RESIDENCY COMPENSATION

Medical residents in the U.S. are compensated at a rate well above the U.S. national wage index. The U.S. average yearly salary is $44,321 USD before taxes with first year residents receiving an average salary of $50,785 USD. In general, not considering the cost of living, residents are compensated the most in the Northeast, the least in the South, and at the average range for the Midwest and West. The average compensation increased 1.0% from 2012 to 2013 and 1.8% from 2013 to 2014.

TABLE 6-M: AVERAGE U.S. RESIDENCY COMPENSATION 2013-14

Years of Training Post-M.D.	Mean in USD	25th Percentile	50th Percentile	75th Percentile
1 year	$50,785	$48,585	$50,214	$52,500
2 years	$52,689	$50,225	$52,048	$54,528
3 years	$54,695	$52,028	$54,024	$56,721
4 years	$56,987	$54,038	$56,380	$59,127
5 years	$59,295	$55,780	$58,599	$61,818
6 years	$62,493	$57,714	$60,972	$64,070
7 years	$63,839	$59,738	$62,905	$66,293
8 years	$66,261	$61,380	$65,738	$69,935

Source: AAMC 2013-2014 Survey of Resident/Fellow Stipend and Benefits Report

It is very important to know how many residency spots are available for each specialty. This can be of particular interest to Caribbean graduates as the availability of specific residencies may limit a student's choice of specialty options. This area should be carefully explored when planning the area of medicine in which the student wants to practice. The average hours that are worked during residency and the time spent on call are important to many when selecting a residency. Residency compensation will differ only slightly depending upon which field is chosen.

TABLE 6-N1: RESIDENCY POSITIONS AND DATA

Residency Program	U.S. Program Spots	Average Hours Per Week
Anesthesiology	1653	59.9
Anatomic Pathology	337	47.4
Dermatology	270	43.3
Diagnostic Radiology	846	51.1
Emergency Medicine	1118	55.5
Family Medicine	2708	64.1
General Surgery	1977	79.9
Internal Medicine	5121	66.1
Neurology	60	61.7
Neurosurgery	32	74.0

Source: Caribbean Medical Schools - A Guide for Canadians and NRMP®)

TABLE 6-N2 RESIDENCY POSITIONS AND DATA

Residency Program	U.S. Program Spots	Average Hours Per Week
Nuclear Medicine	6	45.2
OB/GYN	1120	74.8
Ophthalmology	9	51.8
Orthopedic Surgery	561	67.7
Otolaryngology	42	67.8
Pediatrics	2482	71.4
Physical Med/Rehab	313	51.2
Plastic Surgery	77	64.8
Psychiatry	994	53.6
Radiation Oncology	97	48.5
Urology	62	67.9

Source: Caribbean Medical Schools - A Guide for Canadians and NRMP®)

Chapter 7
Financial Aid

The cost of a Central and South America medical education can be high. The overall cost of the education alone can go as high as $130,000 USD. This often does not include travel, living expenses, fees, books, and other expenses. Each school will want to have proof that a student is able to pay for or finance their education prior to matriculation. Financial aid and scholarships can help to defer some of these expenses but are not guaranteed. Luckily for citizens of the United States, most of the United States educational foreign aid has gone to Caribbean and Central and South America medical schools consistently over the last fifteen years. The National Commission for Medical Education and Accreditation (NCFMEA) exists for the purpose of establishing eligibility requirements to participate in specific loan programs. The Federal Family Education Loan Program (FFELP) is the United States government student loan program that provides Stafford loans.

The salaries of physicians depend upon a number of factors to include the specialty, experience, and the geographical location within the United States where the physician practices. A prospective student should keep in mind that regardless of the study or article that they may read on physician salaries, that salaries change rapidly in today's healthcare environment. All students should become informed and be realistic about how much money they can earn when they graduate. Students need to identify their income range for at least five years. The income that can be earned during the internship and residency is also important. Once the income is identified, the student should take the gross income and reduce it by twenty-five to thirty percent to account for federal, state, social security, and Medicare taxes. The amount left over is what will be left for repayment of the student loans and for living expenses.

When making payments, it is helpful to write checks rather than to use money orders if at all possible when dealing with each school. By doing this, it will be possible to know when the school has processed the application from the date that the check was processed. This will also provide a reliable method of tracking monies received by the various institutions.

HOW MUCH FINANCIAL AID TO ACCEPT

When deciding how much financial aid that a student wants to apply for, many factors must be considered. To begin, students should review all sources of financial support to include parental support, support from relatives, and from friends. For married students, spousal income will be a major source of support. Students should also seek grants or scholarships through companies or corporations, fraternal organizations, and religious groups.

The primary source of payment for medical school will lie with the student and the students' parents. Although most students will prefer to establish independence from their parents, federal regulations require that parental income and assets be considered when granting aid for specific programs. This ensures that the students in the greatest need will be the ones who receive the financial aid.

Students must review their current debts. If student loans have already been taken, can the payments be deferred? If so, will interest be charged while the student is in school? Does the student have a car payment, a mortgage, or credit card debt? Can these balances be reduced or paid off before starting school? Any debt that can be reduced or removed prior to beginning medical school is a plus.

United States students should also review their credit rating. Look at the rating before, not after, enrollment. Students will have a difficult time obtaining student loans if they have ever had a bankruptcy, defaulted on a student loan, or had a tax lien or a civil judgment entered against them. Many lenders will refuse to grant student loans if the student habitually pays their accounts slowly. The credit reporting agencies will charge a fee to obtain a credit report although some companies may allow one free copy each year. Anyone who has been denied credit in the last 60 days is entitled to a free credit report.

The credit criteria used to approve student loans will include the following:

- Absence of negative credit

- No bankruptcies, repossessions, foreclosures, open judgments, or charge-offs

- No prior educational loan defaults unless paid in full or making satisfactory progress in repayment

- Absence of excessive past due accounts

- No 30, 60 or 90-day delinquencies on consumer loans or revolving charge accounts within the past two years.

Table 7-A: CREDIT REPORTING AGENCIES

NAME	ADDRESS	TELEPHONE
EQUIFAX (www.equifax.com)	Information Service Center P.O. Box 740241 Atlanta, GA 30374-0241	1-800-685-1111
TRANS UNION CORPORATION (www.transunion.com)	Consumer Disclosure Center P.O. Box 1000 Chester, PA 19022	1-800-916-8800
EXPERIAN (www.experian.com)	Consumer Assistance Center P.O. Box 2104 Allen TX, 75013-0949	1-888-EXPERIAN (1-888-397-3742)

FINANCIAL AID APPLICATION PROCESS

Colleges that participate in United States financial aid programs will determine the student's financial need by using the Free Application for Federal Student Aid (FAFSA). For these schools, this application is required in order to qualify for financial assistance programs. Students will need the title IV school code for the school to which they have been accepted. The FAFSA should be submitted upon acceptance and a renewal FAFSA application can be submitted if the student has completed this form in previous years. The FAFSA can now be completed via the Internet. Students will receive a Student Aid Report (SAR) approximately four weeks after the application has been filed. The need determined from this report will determine the student's ability to help pay for their education. Parental information is required regardless of the age of the student. Students will be required to reapply for financial aid each year as financial situations and earnings may differ from year to year.

Students must plan a realistic expense budget. Many schools provided budgets for their students, but these should be regarded as guidelines only. Students will have different lifestyles, needs, and wants; and the finances required by individual students can vary greatly.

Table 7-B: Monthly Student Budget

LIVING EXPENSES	ACTUAL - 20___	PROJECTED - 20___
Rent/mortgage/housing		
Utilities: Gas/oil		
Electricity		
Water		
Telephone		
Groceries: Food		
Household supplies		
Transportation: subway/bus		
Gasoline		
Car Maintenance		
Other:_____		
Savings		
Credit Cards		
Insurance: Health		
Life		
Auto		
Entertainment: Meals out		

Movies/concerts/theater		
Health club, etc.		
Personal: clothes/laundry		
Grooming(e.g. haircuts)		
Other:_____		
Miscellaneous:		
MONTHLY LIVING BUDGET		
1st and 2nd year students multiply the BUDGET by 9*; 3rd and 4th year students multiply the budget by 12.		

Original Source: Philadelphia College of Osteopathic Medicine

Table 7-C: Yearly Student Budget

EDUCATIONAL EXPENSES	ACTUAL - 20____	PROJECTED - 20____
Tuition		
Fees		
Books		
Supplies		
Special Equipment		
Other:_____		
TOTAL EDUCATIONAL EXPENSES:		
TOTAL LIVING EXPENSES:		
TOTAL LIVING AND EDUCATIONAL EXPENSES:		
INCOME/RESOURCES:		
Money from: Savings:		
Parents/Spouse:		
Work-Study:		

Other Work:		
Scholarships/Grants:		
Loans: Stafford Subsidized:		
Stafford unsubsidized:		
Federal Perkins Loan:		
Primary Care Loan:		
Alternative Loan:		
TOTAL INCOME/RESOURCES:		
INCOME (minus) EXPENSES:		

Original Source: Philadelphia College of Osteopathic Medicine

LOANS

Many schools offer supplemental loans, which may provide for some or all of the funds needed for medical school attendance. These loans are offered at terms and conditions that generally have higher interest rates and fees than government sponsored loans. Eligibility requirements, terms and conditions, and credit criteria vary with available programs and can frequently change.

Every bank will charge a fee when a student obtains a student loan. The fee covers an origination fee and a guarantee fee. The bank retains the origination fee and the guarantee fee is sent to the agency that guarantees or insures the loan. Because banks compete for business, they will rarely charge the maximum fees allowed by law. An example is if $20,000 is borrowed with a 3% fee, the student will receive $19,400. If $20,000 is borrowed with a 7% fee, the student will receive $18,600. When repayment begins, the principal is what is repaid, not the net. Interest is also computed on the principal and not the net.

Repayment on the student loans will begin after the residency is completed and after the grace period has expired. Most repayment terms will span 10, 20, or even 30 years. Longer repayment terms will result in the student paying more interest. Many private loans are available from multiple sources. The most common and utilized resources are described below.

FINANCIAL SOURCES

Federal Unsubsidized Stafford Loan Program (SLS) - This is a variable interest loan that provides $10,000 USD per academic year with a cumulative maximum of $73,500 USD. The student is responsible for all interest that accrues during the life of the loan and the interest is capped at 8.25%. Unpaid interest is capitalized when the loan enters the repayment period. Interest may be paid while the student is in school or deferred until graduation, or until a student becomes enrolled less than half-time. Students have up to 10 years to repay with $50 USD minimum monthly payments. To be eligible, students must be enrolled in at least half-time and the loan is based on the cost of attendance less other aid received. SLS is available to U.S. citizens, U.S. nationals, and permanent U.S. residents.

Federal Subsidized Stafford Loan Program - This is a variable interest loan that provides $8,500 USD per academic year up to a cumulative maximum of

$65,000 USD. No interest accrues while the student is in school or during the grace period. Interest is not capitalized and interest is capped at 8.25%. Students have up to 10 years to repay with $50 USD minimum monthly payments. To be eligible, students must be enrolled at least half-time and the loan is based on financial need. Stafford is available to U.S. citizens, U.S. nationals, or permanent U.S. residents.

Canadian Student Loan - Provides $105.00 CN for each instructional week of study, although some variations in funds apply in different provinces. The Ministry of Education of each province approves these loans. The Canadian government subsidizes the interest while the student is in school.

International Health Education Loan Program (TERI) - Provides $15,000 USD per academic year. The loan is non-need based and requires a co-signer and/or a co-borrower. It is available to U.S. citizens or permanent residents but can also be received by Canadian residents who can provide a credit-worthy U.S. co-signer.

Veterans Benefits - Dependent upon each individual case. Veterans should contact the Department of Veterans' Affairs.

Post-9/11 GI Bill – Provides finances for educational and housing to veterans who have completed a minimum of 90 days of service after September 10, 2001. Only those who have received an honorable discharge are eligible. Up to 36 months of benefits are available. Currently, tuition and fees of $18,077 USD per academic year can be paid with a monthly housing allowance of $1,368 USD, and a yearly book allowance of $1,000 USD.

International Select Alternative Loan - Provides up to $35,000 USD per year for U.S. students and $20,000 USD for two semesters of full-time study for Canadian residents. This loan is designed to cover the difference between the attendance cost and the amount that the Stafford loans or other loans provide. This loan is available to U.S. citizens or permanent residents and Canadian students with good credit histories. The Educational Finance Group (EFG) administers this loan.

Nation-wide Loan Program - Students may borrow up to $50,000 USD per year depending on credit history and the income of the applicant and co-signers. Official loan applications are directed through the university and not directly to loan agents. Applications can only be processed after students have been admitted to the university. The credit and income based nature of the loan does not guarantee funding.

Key Education Loan - Key Education Resources provides products and services through the Key Bank, USA. Loans are available from Key Education Resources to include the MedAchiever loan and the MedAchiever Residency Travel and Relocation loan. The Key Alternative loan and the Alternative DEAL's Best BET (Board Exam and Travel) loans are also available.

MedAchiever Loan - Provides annually up to the cost of education minus other forms of financial aid. The minimum loan amount is $500 USD and no payments are required during school and for the 48 months after graduation. This loan is offered through the Key Bank, USA and is available for U.S. citizens and permanent residents.

MedCAP Alternative Loan for Health Professionals – Provides up to a maximum life-time limit of $250,000 USD to be combined with existing debt up to the $250,000 USD limit. There is no yearly maximum on the amount that can be taken out. The program is designed for health professionals and can be used to cover the cost of education, books, lab supplies, tuition, computers, and living expenses. Repayment can be delayed up to 60 months for MD and DO students. No application, origination, or early repayment fees apply. Students may select a fixed or variable interest option. The majority of students are able to qualify without a cosigner.

ED-Invest Foreign Medical School Student Loan Program – Designed for international medical school programs and students. This program provides funding in variable amounts and at varying interest rates for select applicants.

Chapter 8
International and Island Life

Island and international life can be a challenge. Individual countries have unique and specific histories. Some are French, some are British, many are Spanish, others are Dutch, and some are independent. The history of the country plays a large part in the individual personality, but many similarities between the islands and countries also exist. Life on the islands or in a Central and South American country is unlike life in the United States and will be an experience to remember. Service is slow and power outages are common. No one will be in a hurry and deadlines do not seem to exist. This can be a difficult adjustment when coming from a society that has to have everything now and in a hurry. Many of the staples of the American diet are not available throughout the regions, although some medical schools have cafeterias with American style menus. Items that are available are overpriced and in short supply. Even though one is attending a medical school, medical care, and particularly medical facilities, are often sub-par. If a true illness or injury arises, it may be desirable to leave the island.

Many countries, particularly those on islands will, however, offer palm-tree lined white sand beaches and blue waters. Many locations have towering mountain peaks, dense tropical jungles, volcanoes, and hot springs. The citizens are generally friendly and helpful particularly when they become acquainted with the students. The crime rate is generally low and almost nonexistent on some islands. Most of the beaches have escaped modern monster resorts that take over miles of beachfront. Diving and snorkeling spots abound and yield some of the most pristine and beautiful sights in the world. Old shipwrecks are common and within easy reach of divers. Bonefish, permit, mutton, snapper, tarpon, shark, jack, and barracuda provide for fishing excursions, and golf is available on some islands

It will be very important to understand the individual laws of each country that a student will be going to. On some islands, women are not allowed to wear bathing suits, on other islands, nude bathing is allowed. In Barbados, it is against the law for anyone except the military to wear camouflage clothing of any type including children. In Curacao, prostitution is legal. Many other unique laws and customs can be found throughout Central and South America and the Caribbean Region.

Climate - The climate throughout the regions varies little from one area to the next with an average year round temperature between 75° and 80° Fahrenheit (24°-27° Celsius). Humidity is generally low and trade winds keep the islands cool on the coast though summer days can be hot. Short rainstorms are frequent so rain gear and an umbrella should be brought to the locations. During the hurricane season every fall, all island inhabitants should pay attention to the weather carefully. Insect repellant and vitamin B should be brought to the areas as mosquitoes are prevalent throughout the islands and jungle areas and this can be overwhelming at times.

Dress - Casual clothes such as t-shirts, shorts, and walking shoes are typically worn on a daily basis. Outer and under garments made out of a cotton blend tend to be more comfortable than those with synthetic blends due to the climate. At least one formal outfit, slacks and a shirt for men, and a skirt and a dress for women, should be brought to the schools for formal presentations and other special events. Sunglasses and a hat are also useful items to bring. Some regions will have dress requirements, particularly for women. Bathing suits are not allowed in some villages, and women are required to wear skirts in all public places in a few areas. This should be investigated beforehand so that there will be no surprises.

Banking and currency - The official currency differs for many of the countries and the exchange rate can fluctuate according to world money markets. The currency of each country is given with each school listing. United States currency should be exchanged directly in purchasing goods and services, as banks will usually charge a small fee to exchange United States currency. Students are advised to arrive with adequate spending money in travelers' checks and it is important to keep travelers' checks in a waterproof pouch, as they are considered void if they get wet.

United States dollars are widely used and accepted nearly everywhere. Credit cards are also often accepted but not nearly as often as cash. As the exchange rates differ, students should make sure what monetary system purchases are quoted in. It is not uncommon to be overcharged in international dollars when one assumed that they were paying in United States dollars. This is especially important when using credit cards. Cash prices are often lower than credit card purchases and most prices are not set in stone. Haggling is common and accepted.

Health insurance - Students should obtain an international health insurance policy from their country of residence. Medical evacuation insurance is also recommended in the case of a serious medical problem. Most schools will offer healthcare for minor health problems but major problems will not be covered.

Transportation - Most students can easily navigate the areas on foot and by bicycle. Other transportation is best achieved using taxis and minibuses, which are available throughout the areas. Personal vehicles can be shipped over, but this will cost a considerable amount. Many students purchase motorbikes and temporary licenses are usually required from the country's traffic department for these. Also, locals will frequently give rides to students as they begin to know them. Many students comment that, after their first year, they can get around just about anywhere this way. Driving is on the right hand side of the road in some areas and on the left on others.

Mail - Regular mail can be slow and will take approximately two weeks to arrive and to travel to its destination. AIRMAIL and Federal Express are available and generally provide the most reliable and best service. Express mail is available in some locales and can arrive within three days in some areas.

Taxes and tipping - If staying in hotels, government room taxes will usually be added at a rate of 5-8%. This tax will automatically be added to your bill. A service charge of 10% to 15% can also be added to some bills. Tipping is voluntary and a rate of 10% is acceptable, more if service is exceptional. For taxis and guides, tip at your own discretion.

Departure tax - A departure tax is often required when leaving the country. This will average around $10 USD. This tax must usually be paid in cash or travelers' checks. Students entering from countries other than the United States can also be charged a security fee which averages at $1 USD.

Firearms - It is illegal to take firearms and ammunition into or out of nearly every country. Do not, therefore, even attempt this.

Animals - Animals must be accompanied by a certificate of freedom from infection and contagious disease by a veterinarian not more than 48 hours prior to shipment. Animals must also have rabies certification not less than one month, or more than six months, prior to departure. The animal must be free of open wounds. Dogs must have a valid certification of vaccination against distemper, parvovirus, infectious canine hepatitis, and leptospirosis. Animals may be required to be revaccinated against rabies on arrival if certifications are deemed unsatisfactory.

Customs - United States residents are permitted a $400 per person USD (or $1,100 USD per family) duty-free tax exemption upon returning to the United States and can also bring back one quart of alcohol and 200 cigarettes duty-free. International customs vary greatly for those returning to countries other than the United States.

Water - Most homes and businesses use cisterns to collect rainwater for drinking and home use. Tap water is, therefore, usually potable with no ill effects. In severe droughts cisterns may run dry making bottled water advisable. Students should be aware of the need to conserve water during the dry season especially on smaller islands.

Electricity - Electrical current is available in several different voltages. Voltage of 110 volts just as in the United States is common, but can range from 110-130 volts, and also is available in 220 volts in some locales. Cycles can vary also but are found usually between 50 and 60 cycles. Most United States appliances that operate on 60 cycles will work fine except for items like hair dryers, irons, and some battery charging equipment which may overheat if used for an extended time period. European appliances usually will not work without adapters. The student should bring AC transformers and adapters that are needed to the school. Power outages are common throughout the regions even when storms are not active.

Communications - Voice communications are available at all locations through local telephone companies. Most schools have, or are in the process of installing, high-speed wireless networks. Telephone service can be easily interrupted in many areas as power outages and storms arise. Most locations have worldwide direct dialing.

Employment - Employment opportunities for students and their spouses are extremely limited. A work visa must be granted and is required for foreigners to work in the countries; these are rarely granted. Exceptions can be made for individuals with healthcare licenses and for areas of particular need.

Immigration requirements - Immigration requirements are in place and the countries require several items prior to arrival. Many areas require either an entrance fee or an entrance deposit when entering the country that can range from hundreds to thousands of dollars. Some variation in what is needed will depend on the specific country. Accepted students should be prepared to provide the following:

- A health certificate to include a current list of immunizations and a TB (Tuberculin) test
- Proof of being HIV negative
- VDRL or RPR (serologic test for syphilis)
- A letter of good conduct from the local police department where the student lives
- A valid passport

- Color 2x2 passport sized photographs - between four to eight are usually required.
- Proof of a roundtrip plane ticket

Chapter 9

The Schools

International medical schools that base their educational curriculum on the model used by United States and provide instruction in English are listed below. Medical school locations are listed based on physiographic location and divided by those listed in this publication and those in the Greater and Lesser Antilles described in the AMRCB® Caribbean Medical School publication. Islands that lie on the South American geologic shelf are listed in the Central and South American publication and include Aruba, Bonaire, Curacao, and Trinidad and Tobago. Other medical schools may exist in these areas as well but are not listed in this publication if instruction is not in English or if the educational curriculum does not follow U.S. standards.

Medical schools listed in this publication include:

CENTRAL AND SOUTH AMERICA
(Caribbean Region)

CENTRAL AMERICA

Belize: pg. # 110

- American Global University School of Medicine
- Avicina Medical Academy
- Central America Health Sciences University Belize Medical College
- Grace University School of Medicine
- Hope University School of Medicine

Central and South American Medical Schools - Caribbean Region

- InterAmerican Medical University
- Medical University of the Americas
- St. Luke's University School of Medicine
- St. Matthew's University School of Medicine
- Washington University of Health and Sciences

Panama: pg. #190

- Columbus University School of Medicine and Health Sciences

SOUTH AMERICA
Aruba: pg. #204

- Aureus University School of Medicine
- Xavier University School of Medicine

Bonaire: pg. #224

- St. James School of Medicine – Bonaire

Curacao: pg. #236

- Avalon University School of Medicine
- Caribbean Medical University School of Medicine
- St. Martinus University Faculty of Medicine

Guyana: pg. #272

- American International School of Medicine
- GreenHeart Medical University School of Medicine
- Texila American University College of Medicine
- University of Guyana Faculty of Health Sciences

Central and South American Medical Schools - Caribbean Region

<u>Trinidad and Tobago:</u> pg. #314

- University of the West Indies Faculty of Medicine - St. Augustine

The following medical schools are described in the AMRCB® publication entitled: Caribbean Medical Schools – Greater and Lesser Antilles - Based on a U.S. Curriculum – The Complete Guide to Medical Schools, Acceptance Criteria, and International Life. The third edition was released in 2014, ISBN 978-1500419042

Anguilla:

- Saint James School of Medicine – Anguilla

Antigua and Barbuda:

- American University of Antigua College of Medicine
- University of Health Sciences Antigua School of Medicine

Barbados:

- American University of Barbados School of Medicine
- University of the West Indies - Barbados Faculty of Medical Sciences

Cayman Islands:

- St. Matthew's University School of Medicine

Dominica:

- All Saints University School of Medicine
- Ross University School of Medicine

Dominican Republic:

- Universidad Iberoamericana (UNIBE) School of Medicine

Grenada:

- St. George's University School of Medicine

Jamaica:

- All American Institute of Medical Sciences
- University of the West Indies Faculty of Medical Sciences - Kingstown

Montserrat:

- Seoul Central College of Medicine
- University of Science, Arts, & Technology (USAT) Faculty of Medicine
- Vanguard University School of Medicine

Saba:

- Saba University School of Medicine

Saint Kitts and Nevis:

- Burnett International University School of Medicine and Health Sciences
- Grace University School of Medicine
- International University of the Health Sciences
- Medical University of the Americas
- Milik University
- Saint Theresa's Medical University
- University of Medicine and Health Sciences
- Windsor University School of Medicine

Saint Lucia:

- American International Medical University School of Medicine
- Atlantic University School of Medicine
- College of Medicine and Health Sciences
- Destiny University School of Medicine and Health Sciences
- International American University College of Medicine
- Spartan Health Sciences University School of Medicine
- St. Helen University School of Medicine

- St. Mary's School of Medicine
- Washington Medical Sciences Institute

Saint Martin:

- American University of the Caribbean School of Medicine
- University of Sint Eustatius School of Medicine

Saint Vincent and the Grenadines:

- All Saints University College of Medicine
- American University of St. Vincent School of Medicine
- Kingstown Medical College
- Saint James School of Medicine - St. Vincent and the Grenadines
- Trinity School of Medicine

American Global University School of Medicine

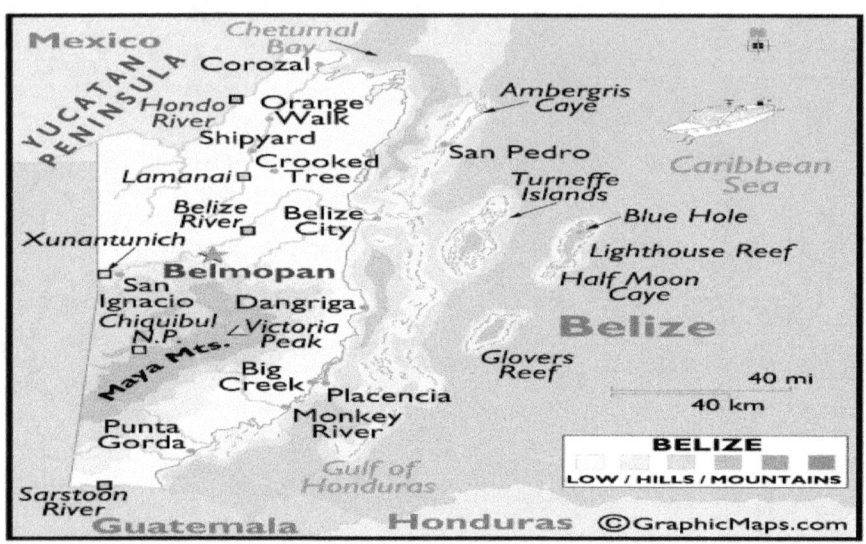

AMRCB® QUICK REFERENCE
American Global University School of Medicine

Year Founded	2005	Currency	BZD
On-Campus Housing	Yes	Airport Code	BZE
Pre-Medical Program	Yes	Time Zone	CST (GMT/UTC-6)
MCAT® Required	No	Electricity	110 V
Official Language	English	Driving Side	Right

American Global University School of Medicine

Belize

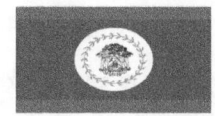

Malik J. Soudah, M.D. – President
Shakel Henson, M.P.H., M.D. – Clinical Medicine

CONTACT INFORMATION:

U.S. Admissions Office
American Global University
c/o Med Serve International
118 Graceland Blvd, Suite 311
Columbus, OH 43214 U.S.A.
Email: info@agusm.org

Campus Address
American Global University
Phillip Goldson Road
Ladyville, Belize
Phone: 011-501-226-2682

U.K. Mailing Office
Med One International
American Global University
SOM, Suite 62
2 Landsdowne Crescent
Bournemouth, BH1 1SA, U.K
Email: operations@agusm.org

General Information
Email: admissions@agusm.org
Phone: 1-866-990-2248
Fax: 1-312-873-3815
Website: http://www.agusm.org/

GENERAL INFORMATION:

The American Global University School of Medicine (AGUSM) was founded in 2005 with the first medical school class starting in 2006. The school was initially opened in San Pedro, Ambergris Caye, but moved to Ladyville near the international airport after the campus was expanded in 2011. AGUSM seeks to train students from the U.S., Europe, and the international community in training scientifically and clinically competent and compassionate physicians. The school desires to educate and inspire scholars and future educators. The USMLE® Step 1 first time pass rate is 87% with average step one scores of 221. The maximum class size is 60 students.

The campus is a multi-media A-class complex with classrooms and lecture halls, offices, a computer lab, laboratories, student lounge, fitness club, and library. The campus complex can support up to 2000 active students. AGUSM has an additional campus in the European Union that opened in 2010. On-campus and off-campus student housing is available for an average cost of $500 USD per month.

The curriculum is modeled after the United States and AUGSM strives to find the most effective and efficient way of educating new physicians. Problem-based learning is utilized as well as case studies, question banks, and lectures. The school has affiliated with multiple teaching hospitals in the United States. Dual Master of Business Administration (M.B.A.) degree programs are available with Davenport University and Walden University. The school operates under a rolling admissions system with classes starting in January, May, and September each year.

AGUSM is not currently certified by the American Medical Residency Certification Board (AMRCB®). AGUSM is listed by the International Medical Education Directory (IMED), the World Health Organization (WHO), and the Medical Council of Canada (MCC). AGUSM is chartered and licensed by the Government of Belize. Students are eligible for ECFMG® certification.

CURRICULUM:

Pre-Medical Program

The pre-medical program is conducted over three semesters of 16 weeks each and students can enter the program yearly at any semester. The instruction takes place on the AGUSM campus in Belize. The program is designed to provide a firm foundation for the advanced study of medical sciences. Upon completion, students with a minimum GPA of 2.5 and who pass the Premedical Science Post Examination (PSPE) can directly apply to the AGUSM M.D. program. The class size is relatively small at 20 students as the majority of applicants area accepted directly into the M.D. program.

Pre-Medical Curriculum

Pre-Med Semester I	Pre-Med Semester II	Pre-Med Semester III
Foundation Biology I	Foundation Biology II	Foundation Biology III
General Chemistry I	General Chemistry II	General Chemistry III
General Physics I	General Physics II	General Physics III
Organic Chemistry I	Organic Chemistry II	Psychology II
English I	English II	Human Anatomy
Mathematics I	Psychology I	Mathematics II

M.D. Program

The curriculum is conducted over a four-year program consisting of 11 semesters. The Basic Sciences are conducted over the first four semesters, with a fifth "bridge" semester in place which transitions students into the five Clinical Science rotations. Patient exposure begins in the first year.

Basic Sciences

The Basic Sciences are conducted over four semesters which span 16 weeks each and are taught on the Belize campus. The fifth semester which is designed as a bridge to the Clinical Medicine program is taught in the U.S.A. in either Orlando, Florida or Chicago, Illinois. A dedicated USMLE® preparation program is built into the Basic Science curriculum and the school offers an elective USMLE® review course in offered in Belize or in Chicago, Illinois.

Basic Science Curriculum

Semester I	Semester II	Semester III	Semester IV	Semester V
Histology and Cell Biology and Lab	Behavioral Science	Microbiology	Pharmacology	Intro to Clinical Medicine
Gross Anatomy with Lab	Physiology	Immunology	Systemic Pathology II with Lab	Physical Diagnosis
Embryology	NeuroAnatomy	General Pathology I with Lab	Biostatistics and Epidemiology	USMLE® Review
Biochemistry	Nutrition	Medical Genetics	USMLE® Review	
Medical terminology	USMLE® Review	Medical and Legal Ethics		
USMLE® Review		USMLE® Review		

Clinical Sciences

The Clinical clerkships are conducted over 72 weeks for semesters six through eleven and can occur in the United States, United Kingdom, and the Caribbean region. Many sites are available that allow the student to complete all 72 weeks in one location.

Clinical Science Curriculum

Required – 48 weeks (Semester VI-IX)		Electives and Selectives – 24 weeks (Semester X and XI)	
Internal Medicine	12 - weeks	Selectives	
Surgery	12 - weeks	Cardiology	4 - weeks
Pediatrics	6 - weeks	Neurology	4 - weeks
OB/GYN	6 - weeks	Emergency Medicine	4 - weeks
Psychiatry	6 - weeks	Electives	
Family Medicine	6 - weeks	Student Choice	12 - weeks

Grading

Students are promoted from one semester to the next after passing all courses for that semester and achieve graduation after satisfactorily meeting all performance standards. Computerized test scoring and online grading reports are utilized. The Dean promotes a student into the Clinical Science clerkship program only after completing all of the Basic Science program requirements and passing USMLE® Step 1. Students are required to take USMLE® Step 1 within four months of completing the Basic Sciences. To be eligible for graduation, all students must successfully complete each of the following: all required coursework; pass USMLE® Step 1 in three or less attempts; and pass USMLE® Step 2 CS and CK in three or less attempts.

ENTRANCE REQUIREMENTS:

Pre-Medical Program

Applicants must have a high school diploma or equivalent and SAT or ACT scores must be submitted. SAT scores are expected to be 1200 or greater and ACT scores must be at least 26. TOEFL® scores must be at least 213 and IELTS™ scores should be 6.0 or higher. Two letters of recommendation are required. Accepted applicants will usually have a high school GPA of 2.7 or greater. Students who have lower GPA scores should have strong letters of recommendation in order to demonstrate that they have the motivation needed to study medicine. Applicants will be directed in the appropriate premedical semester according to their academic background.

M.D. Program

The minimum requirement for admission is 90 semester hours of college level courses. A baccalaureate degree or equivalent is preferred but not required. College work must include the following (lab work is required nearly universally even when not specifically stated):

- General Biology or Zoology – one academic year
- General Chemistry – one academic year
- Organic Chemistry – one academic year
- General Physics – one academic year
- English – one academic semester
- Mathematics (Calculus, Computer Science, or Statistics) – one academic semester

International applicant from countries other than the United States should have completed prerequisites comparable to those described above. The MCAT® is optional.

SELECTION FACTORS:

The school has an open admissions system and advanced standing is considered for transfer applicants. AGUSM seeks to identify future physicians that will positively contribute to the community of healthcare providers. Students are evaluated individually and selected based on social maturity, intellect, educational, and social backgrounds. Students are sought that have critical judgment, maturity, problem-solving skills, personal integrity, and the ability to study independently. Students are expected to have effective observation skills, communication skills, motor skills, and intellectual and conceptual abilities. The Admissions Committee considers the major area of study, the course load, and the difficulty in the courses taken. The personal essay is an applicant's opportunity to demonstrate their interest in medicine, goals in pursuing medical training, and their individual attributes that qualify the student to become a physician.

Although the MCAT® is optional, students who have taken the test should report their scores. For applicants that have not taken the MCAT®, or for those that have GPA's that are not strong, the Admissions Committee expects strong letters of recommendation. A minimum GPA of 2.5 is required for admission. A TEOFL® score of 550 on the paper test or 231 on the computer test, or an IELTS™ score of 6.0 is required for applicants whose primary language is not English. Preference will be given to applicants with higher GPA's and those who have completed a Bachelor's degree or higher. Applications from non-North American students are considered and evaluated on an individual basis. Once all required admissions documents are received, a phone interview may be scheduled to evaluate a student's overall character and motivation to study medicine. The interview will be just as important as college grades and test scores. Applicants will be notified within two to three weeks of the admissions decision. There is no application deadline as the school operates under a rolling admissions system with classes starting in January, May, and September.

TUITION AND FINANCIAL AID:

Application Fee: $100 USD (non-refundable)

Enrollment Fee to secure acceptance: $1000 USD (credited toward tuition)

Registration Fee: $500 USD

Tuition for Pre-Medical Sciences (semesters 1-3): $5,195 USD per semester

Tuition for Basic Sciences (semester 1-5): $6,195 USD per semester

Tuition for Clinical Sciences (semesters 6-11): $8,295 USD per semester

Graduation Fee: $1200 USD

Student Government Fee: $40 USD per semester

Laboratory Fee: $300-500 USD per semester

Other fees such as student and administrative may apply

Scholarships, merit-based awards, private student loans, tuition deferment, payment plans, and partial or full tuition waivers are available. United States Federal student loans are not available at this time. Five full scholarships are offered yearly to citizens of Belize and all other citizens of Belize receive a tuition discount of 50%.

ooooo

Avicina Medical Academy

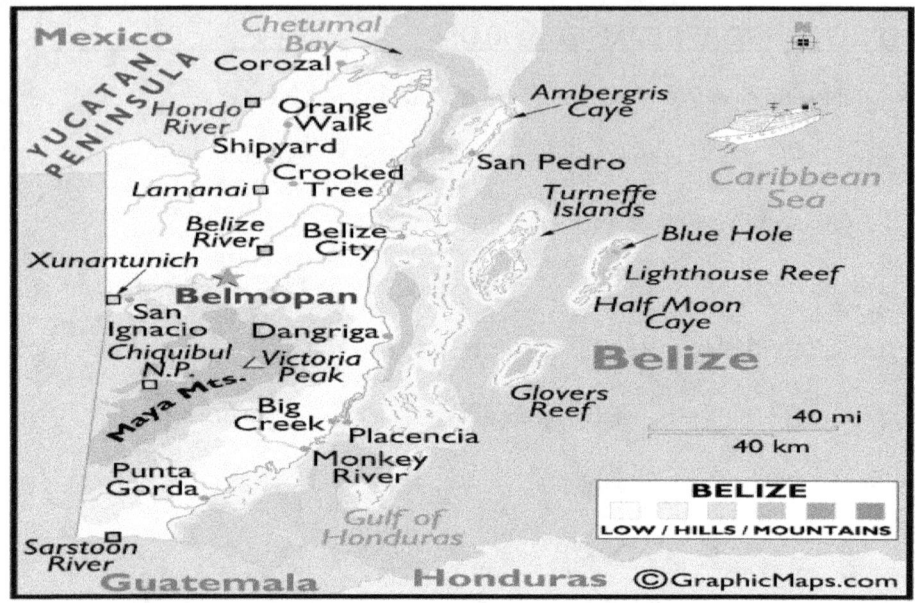

AMRCB® QUICK REFERENCE
Avicina Medical Academy

Year Founded	2012	Currency	BZD
On-Campus Housing	Yes	Airport Code	BZE
Pre-Medical Program	Yes	Time Zone	CST (GMT/UTC-6)
MCAT® Required	No	Electricity	110 V
Official Language	English	Driving Side	Right

Avicina Medical Academy

Belize

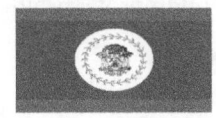

Moneer Avicina Werdeg, M.D. – President
Sakib Khan, M.D. – Dean of Clinical Medicine
Daisy Reyna, N.P., M.S.N. – Dean of Medical Sciences

CONTACT INFORMATION:

U.S. Admissions Office
Avicina Medical Academy
10661 S. Roberts Road
Suite 207
Palos Hills, Illinois U.S.A. 60645
E-Mail: info-USA@avicina.bz
Telephone: (708) 600-0902

Campus Address
P.O. Box 621
Emporium Plaza
Belmopan City, Caya District
E-Mail: info-Belize@avicina.bz

Canadian Admissions Office
Avicina Medical Academy
771 Brimley Road
Toronto, Ontario M1C1J7 Canada
Telephone: (416) 568-3137

General Information
Website: http://avicina.bz/
E-Mail: info@avicina.bz
Admissions: (312) 646-0080
Telephone: (501) 822-0292

GENERAL INFORMATION:

Avicina Medical Academy was founded in 2012. The class sizes are small with a maximum number of students set at 25 per class. The mission of the school is to educate and inspire scholars and future leaders to create and disseminate the practice of medicine, sustain and improve health, and to provide outstanding care and service for patients.

The curriculum is modeled after medical education in the United States and was established to guarantee a student passing rate of 100% on the USMLE®. The current pass rate is 93% for USMLE® Step 1 and 90% for USMLE® Step 2. A three month USMLE® Preparation course is utilized in the curriculum. A Pre-Medical program is available as is the traditional 4-year medical curriculum. Active learning is emphasized and small-group learning, self-directed study, lectures, labs, group seminars, and problem-based learning are all utilized.

Student housing is available within walking distance to campus at a rate of $450 USD per month. Off-campus housing is also available and Avicina will aid students in coordinating this. The campus is located in Belmopan directly next to the American embassy. No admissions deadline is in place as the school operates under a rolling admissions system with classes starting in January, April, July, and October.

Avicina is not currently certified by the American Medical Residency Certification Board (AMRCB®). Avicina is listed by the International Medical Education Directory (IMED), the World Health Organization (WHO), and the Medical Council of Canada (MCC). Avicina is chartered and accredited by the

Government and Ministry of Education of Belize. Students are eligible for ECFMG® certification.

CURRICULUM:

Pre-Medical Program

The pre-medical program is conducted over one year spanning four quarters and students can enter the program four times a year in January, April, July, and October. The program is designed for high school graduates or students who have not yet completed the required prerequisite coursework and provides a comprehensive approach to pre-medical training. The instruction takes place on the campus in Belize. Upon completion, students who have completed all courses and maintained attendance of at least 90% can proceed directly to the Avicina M.D. program.

Pre-Medical Curriculum

Pre-Med Quarter I	Pre-Med Quarter II	Pre-Med Quarter III	Pre-Med Quarter IV
Biostatistics	Medical Terminology	Inorganic Chemistry	MCAT Prep
Physics	General Biology	Organic Chemistry	AMAT Prep
Mathematics	Anatomy	Physiology	

M.D. Program

The curriculum is conducted over a four-year program spanning 16 months on the campus in Belize. The entire curriculum can be completed in three years and six months. Patient exposure occurs during the Basic Science rotations. Independent and collaborative learning are expected and encouraged.

Basic Sciences

The Basic Sciences are conducted over the first two years spanning eight quarters on the campus in Belize and focuses on the study of organ systems. The first 15-months focus on the Basic Medical Sciences and the last three months focus on USMLE® Step-1 preparation. A USMLE® PREP course (ACEMLE) is utilized over three months to help in preparing students.

Basic Science Curriculum-Year I

Year I			
Quarter I	Quarter II	Quarter III	Quarter IV
Medical Microanatomy	Medical Genetics	Medical Ethics	Medical Physiology
Medical Neuroanatomy	Medical Biochemistry	Medical Biostatistics	Medical Pathology I
Medical Gross Anatomy	Medical Molecular Biology	Medical Microbiology	

Basic Science Curriculum-Year II

Year I			
Quarter I	Quarter II	Quarter III	Quarter IV
Medical Psychology	Intro to Clinical Medicine	USMLE® Review	USMLE® I
Medical Pathology II	Physical Diagnosis		
Medical Pharmacology			

Clinical Sciences

The Clinical clerkships are conducted over 78 weeks in the U.S. and Canada. Professional development is emphasized and reflective practice is embraced.

Clinical Science Curriculum

Required – 54 weeks		Electives and Selectives – 24 weeks	
Internal Medicine	12 - weeks	Selectives	
OB/GYN	12 - weeks	USMLE® II Study	6 weeks
Surgery	12 - weeks	Electives	
Pediatrics	6 - weeks	Student Choice	18 weeks
Psychiatry	6 - weeks		
Family Medicine	6 - weeks		

Grading

Students are promoted from one semester to the next after passing all courses for that semester and achieve graduation after satisfactorily meeting all performance standards. The Dean promotes a student into the Clinical Science clerkship program only after completing all of the Basic Science program requirements and passing USMLE® Step 1.

ENTRANCE REQUIREMENTS:

Pre-Medical Program

The program is designed for students seeking to enter the M.D. track directly from high school or for students who have not yet completed the required prerequisites. Competitive GPA's are expected. Applicants must have a high school diploma. Students are able to enter the program four times yearly in January, April, July, and October.

M.D. Program

The minimum requirement for admission is completion of prerequisite coursework or the Avicina premedical program. College work should include the following (Lab work is nearly universally expected even when not listed):

- Biology – one academic year
- Chemistry – one academic year
- Organic Chemistry or Biochemistry – one academic year
- Physics – one academic year
- Mathematics or Statistics – one academic year

The MCAT® is not required.

SELECTION FACTORS:

The school has an open admissions system and advanced standing is considered for transfer applicants. Avicina seeks to identify students who are motivated and mature and who demonstrate evidence of character, achievement, and academic excellence. The Admissions Committee recognizes the depth, breadth, and difficulty of the academic program the student has completed and students should have studied some subjects in depth beyond the required prerequisite coursework. Life experience, clinical exposure, and research exposure is viewed favorably. Three letters of recommendation are required and the personal statement should be strong. A diverse student body is sought and applicants from underrepresented populations and countries are encouraged to apply. Applicants will receive an initial interview prior to the submission of documents and a second interview after receipt of all required application materials. Applicants will be notified at the earliest possible date of an admissions decision. There is no application deadline as the school operates under a rolling admission system with classes starting in January, April, July, and October.

TUITION AND FINANCIAL AID:

Application Fee: $100 USD (non-refundable)

Enrollment Fee: $1,000 USD

Tuition for Pre-Medical Sciences (quarters 1-4): $2,200-4,400 USD per quarter

Tuition for Basic Sciences (quarters 1-8): $3,300-5,500 USD per quarter

Tuition for Clinical Sciences (quarters 9-16): $4,400-8,800 USD per quarter

Graduation Fee: $1,000 USD

Other fees such as laboratory, student, and administrative may apply. Textbooks are included in tuition.

Yearly scholarships of up to $25,000 USD are available and are awarded solely based on academic achievement. Private and institutional loans are available. United States Federal student loans are not available at this time.

ooooo

Central American Health Sciences University Belize Medical College

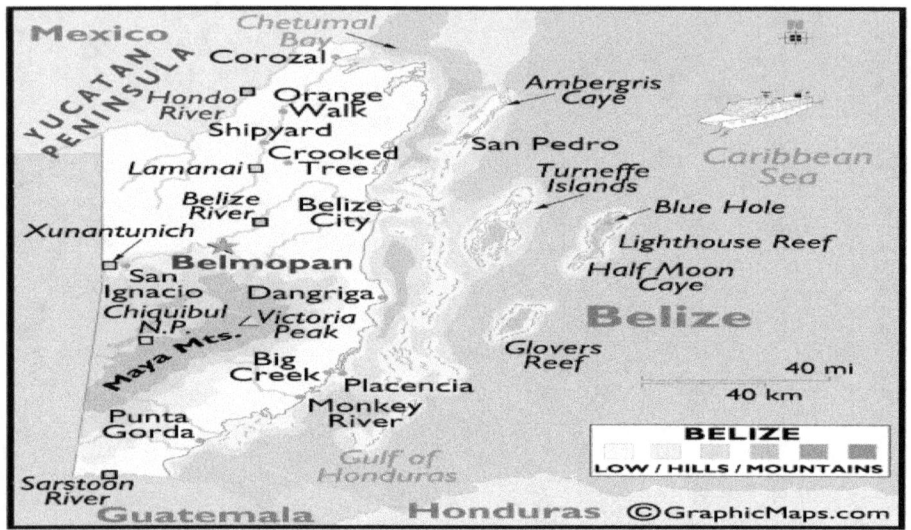

AMRCB® QUICK REFERENCE Central American Health Science University			
Year Founded	1996	Currency	BZD
On-Campus Housing	No	Airport Code	BZE
Pre-Medical Program	Yes	Time Zone	CST (GMT/UTC-6)
MCAT® Required	No	Electricity	110 V
Official Language	English	Driving Side	Right

Central American Health Sciences University Belize Medical College
Belize

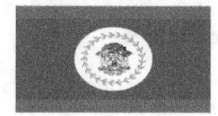

Maurice Modavi, M.D., M.A. – Executive Dean
Murali V. Rudraraju M.D. – Director Special Projects and Development
Virginia Ontiveros – Admissions Coordinator

CONTACT INFORMATION:

U.S. Admissions Office
Central America Health Sciences
University
Belize Medical College
P.O. Box 55996
Washington, D.C. 20040 U.S.A.
Telephone: (877) 523-9687

Campus Address
Central America Health Sciences
University
Belize Medical College
P.O. Box 989
Belize City, Belize
Telephone: +501 (2) 35560
Fax: +501 (2) 35651

General Information
Website: www.cahsu.edu/
E-Mail: admissions@cahsu.edu

GENERAL INFORMATION:

The Central America Health Sciences University Belize Medical College (CAHSU) was founded in 1996. The mission of the school is to promote the health of mankind through education and public service.

The curriculum follows the educational model in the United States. The goal of CAHSU is to provide students with a well-rounded education allowing students to develop into skilled and responsible physicians who are prepared to enter the job market immediately after graduation. The curriculum is designed to teach students normal health and the underlying causes in the physical, chemical, psychological, biologic, and social issues that undermine it. Conferences, laboratory work, and lectures are all utilized.

CAHSU offers the traditional four-year M.D. program and a Pre-Medical program as well. The campus is technologically up-to-date. On-Campus housing is not available. Off-campus student housing ranges from $500-$700 monthly and students typically live in the CAHSU hostel located within 10 minutes of the campus. No admissions deadline is in place as the school operates under a rolling admissions system with classes starting in January, May, and September.

CAHSU is not currently certified by the American Medical Residency Certification Board (AMRCB®). CAHSU is listed by the International Medical Education Directory (IMED), the World Health Organization (WHO), and the General Medical Council (GMC) of the United Kingdom. CAHSU is chartered and accredited by the Government of Belize and approved by the Ministry of Education in Belize. Students are eligible for ECFMG® certification.

CURRICULUM:

Pre-Medical Program

The pre-medical program is conducted over two years on the CAHSU campus in Belize. The program provides a comprehensive approach to pre-medical training. Students are able to completed coursework in Biology, Chemistry, English, Organic Chemistry, Physics, and Mathematics. Upon completion, students can directly apply to the CAHSU M.D. program.

M.D. Program

The curriculum is conducted over a four-year program. The Basic Sciences are conducted over the first five trimesters. The curriculum is designed to provide a high quality medical education and to support and prepare students for active, self-directed learning.

Basic Sciences

The Basic Sciences are conducted over five trimesters over 20 months on the campus in Belize. Students are exposed to clinical encounters during the Basic Sciences at locations in Belize, Mexico, and the United States.

Basic Science Curriculum

Trimester I	Trimester II	Trimester III	Trimester IV	Trimester V
Gross Anatomy	Biochemistry	General Pathology	Gastroenterology	Infectious Disease
Medical Physiology	Microbiology	Pharmacology	Hematology	Molecular Biology
Histology	Neuroanatomy	ENT	Oncology	Cardiology
Embryology	Human Genetics	Respiratory Medicine	Orthopedics	Physical Diagnosis
Biostatistics	Immunology and Allergy	Neurology	Principles of Clinical Medicine	Forensic Medicine
	Behavioral Sciences	Fluids, Electrolytes, and Renal	Radiology	Urology
	Epidemiology and Public Health	Endocrinology	Ophthalmology	Rheumatology
	Nutrition	Dermatology	Pediatrics	
		Legal Medicine and Medical Ethics	Surgery and Orthopedic Surgery	
		Tropical Medicine and Parasitology	Obstetrics and Gynecology	
		Psychiatry	Systemic Pathology	
		Anesthesiology	Geriatric Medicine	
			Child Abuse and Human Sexuality	

Clinical Sciences

The Clinical clerkships are conducted over 88 weeks and occur in United States, Belize, and Mexico.

Clinical Science Curriculum

Required – 72 weeks		Electives – 16 weeks	
Internal Medicine	12 - weeks	Anesthesiology	Dermatology
OB/GYN	12 - weeks	Clinical Pathology	Emergency Medicine
General Surgery	12 - weeks	Internal Medicine	Neurosurgery
Pediatrics	12 - weeks	Orthopedic Surgery	Pathology
Psychiatry	12 - weeks	Pediatric Surgery	Radiology
Primary Care	12 - weeks	Cardiology	many others

Grading

Students are promoted from one semester to the next after passing all courses for that semester and achieve graduation after satisfactorily meeting all performance standards. The minimum class attendance required is 80% and the minimum grade required is 75 on a 100 point scale. The Dean promotes a student into the Clinical Science clerkship program only after completing all of the Basic Science program requirements. To be eligible for graduation, all students must successfully complete the entire curriculum and satisfactorily meet all other requirements.

Grading Scale

H – 90-100 (Honor)

P – 75-89 (Pass)

F – Less than 75 (Fail)

ENTRANCE REQUIREMENTS:

Pre-Medical Program

Applicants who do not meet the premedical requirements may be placed into the CAHSU Pre-Medical program until the requirements have been completed. Upon completion of the prerequisite coursework, students will be admitted into the medical program. The MCAT® is not required for the Pre-Medical program.

M.D. Program

The minimum requirement for admission is 90 semester hours of college level courses. A baccalaureate degree or equivalent is not required but is recommended. College work must include the following:

- Biology with labs – one academic year
- General Chemistry with labs – one academic year
- Organic Chemistry with labs – one academic year
- Physics with labs – one academic year
- English – one academic year
- Mathematics – one academic year

The MCAT® is not required.

SELECTION FACTORS:

The school has an open admissions system and advanced standing is considered for transfer applicants. Advanced standing is not granted for students who hold Allied Health or other Doctoral degrees. CAHSU welcomes applications equally from male and female students representing all ethnic diversities, particularly those that are under-represented in the medical profession. Applicants are evaluated on many different qualities and not solely on academic merit. The Admissions Committee evaluates a student's commitment to the medical field, undergraduate studies, originality, motivation, and academic record. The personal statement should detail the reasons that the students are pursuing a medical career. Two letters of recommendation are required and letters from a physician and/or college professors are preferred.

The MCAT® is not required. Students who have taken the MCAT® may submit scores for consideration at their own discretion. Applicants who meet admissions criteria may be asked for a personal interview at the discretion of the Admissions Committee. Applicants will be notified within four weeks of an admissions decision. There is no application deadline as the school operates under a rolling admission system with classes starting in January, May, and September.

TUITION AND FINANCIAL AID:

Application Fee: $60 USD (non-refundable)

Payment required to secure acceptance: $2,000 USD (not credited toward tuition)

Tuition for Pre-Medical Sciences: Contact CAHSU

Tuition for Basic Sciences (trimester 1-5): $8,000 USD per trimester

Tuition for Clinical Sciences (trimesters 6-10):

- $9,500 USD per trimester – U.S. hospital
- $8,000 USD per trimester – Mexico and Belize

Other fees such as laboratory, student, administrative, and graduation may apply. Select hospitals used in clinical rotations may require a surcharge.

A limited number of scholarships are available each year. A deferred payment plan is also available. United States Federal student loans are not available at this time.

ooooo

Grace University School of Medicine

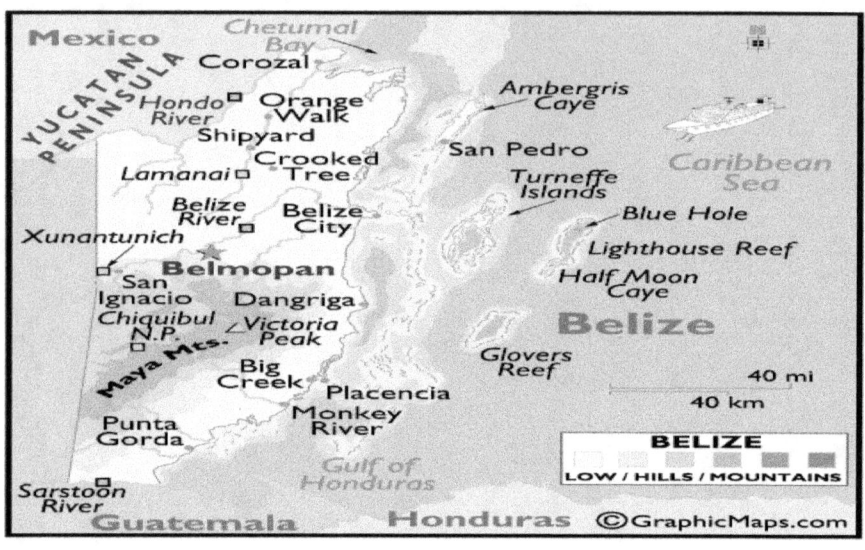

AMRCB® QUICK REFERENCE
Grace University School of Medicine

Years Operated	1984-2004	Currency	BZD
On-Campus Housing	No	Airport Code	BZE
Pre-Medical Program	No	Time Zone	CST (GMT/UTC-6)
MCAT® Required	No	Electricity	110 V
Official Language	English	Driving Side	Right

Grace University School of Medicine
Belize

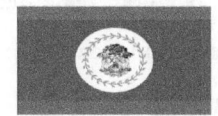

CONTACT INFORMATION:

Prior Campus Address
Grace University School of Medicine
Cades Bay
St. Kitts and Nevis

Prior U.S. Address
Grace Atlantic Admission
23123 State Road 7, Suite 223
Boca Raton, Florida 33428 U.S.A.
Telephone: 561-451-9152
Fax: 561-451-4060

Prior Campus Address
Grace University
3244 Water Reservoir Area
Belmopan, Belize

Contact Information
Telephone: +501 822-2756
Fax: +501 822-2756
Website: http://www.grace-usom.org/
E-Mail: admissions@grace-usom.org

GENERAL INFORMATION:

Grace University School of Medicine (GUSM) was founded in 1984 by J.P. McNaughton-Louden, M.D. upon traditional Christian principles. GUSM operated in St. Kitts and Nevis from 1984 to 1999. In 2000, the medical school signed a memorandum of understanding with the Government of Belize to move operations to Belize. Grace University was granted a ten year operating period on

Belize at that time. This memorandum of understanding was terminated by the government of Belize on December 17th, 2004. The school is not actively operating or instructing students at the time of this publication.

The curriculum was based on a four-year program modeled after the U.S. medical education system. The school offered a Doctorate in Behavioral Sciences as well as the M.D. degree while in operation. The majority of students studied on the campuses in St. Kitts and Nevis and Belize, although some exceptional students received instruction at Cambridge University in England. No official affiliation existed between GUSM and Cambridge University however.

GUSM is not currently certified by the American Medical Residency Certification Board (AMRCB®). GUSM is not listed by the International Medical Education Directory (IMED) or the World Health Organization (WHO) as active at the time of this publication.

CURRICULUM:

M.D. Program

GUSM utilized a systems-based approach to medical education and was one of the first schools to implement this. Lectures were replaced in favor of clinically oriented seminars where students were motivated to learn through active discussion of patient problems. GUSOM's curriculum was designed using 8 modules spanning 11 weeks each during the Basic Sciences with the Clinical Sciences taking place over the last two years. The curriculum was traditionally completed within four years.

Basic Sciences

The first three modules were designed to provide groundwork needed in the remaining five modules. The remaining five modules provide detailed study on each system of the human body covering clinical presentation, function, and dysfunction. The basic sciences were completed in the first two years.

Basic Science Curriculum

Module I	Module II	Module III
Gross Anatomy	Biochemistry and Nutrition	Pathology
Histology and Cell Biology	Physiology	Epidemiology and Preventative Medicine
Embryology	Immunology	Microbiology
Neuroanatomy	Pharmacology	Behavioral Science
Medical Imaging	Molecular Engineering	Intro to Clinical Medicine

Clinical Sciences

The Clinical Science program spanned 88 weeks. Students completed their junior and senior years of clinical training at GUSM affiliated hospitals in several locales. Students could complete all of their clinical rotations in the United States if that was their intention.

Clinical Science Curriculum

Required – 50 weeks		Selectives – 38 weeks	
Internal Medicine	12 - weeks	Selectives – 16 weeks	
Surgery	12 - weeks	Emergency Medicine	4 – weeks
Pediatrics	8 - weeks	Radiology	4 – weeks
OB/GYN	8 - weeks	Neurology	4 – weeks
Psychiatry	6 - weeks	Pathology	4 – weeks
Family Medicine	4 - weeks	Electives – 22 weeks	

Grading

Students were promoted from one semester to the next after passing all courses for that semester and achieved graduation after satisfactorily meeting all performance standards. All examinations were performance based. The Dean promoted a student into the Clinical Science clerkship program only after completing all of the Basic Science program requirements and passing USMLE® Step 1. To be eligible for graduation, students must have successfully completed all curriculum requirements, examinations, and have obtained approval of the Dean.

Grades were distributed as follows:

    H (Honors): 90%-100%

    P (Pass): 70%-89%

    F (Fail): below 70%

ENTRANCE REQUIREMENTS:

M.D. Program

The minimum requirement for admission was 90 semester hours of college level courses. A baccalaureate degree or equivalent was preferred with preference given to applicants with baccalaureate degrees. College work must have included the following:

- General Biology with labs – one academic year
- General Chemistry with labs – one academic year
- Organic Chemistry with labs – one academic year
- General Physics with labs – one academic year
- English – one academic year
- Calculus – one academic year
- Foreign Language – one academic year
- Humanities – one academic year

Although not required, the MCAT® was highly recommended.

SELECTION FACTORS:

Students were selected based upon several factors. Applicants must have demonstrated compassion, maturity, considerable academic achievement, motivation, and mental and physical stamina. The ability to learn in an increasingly complex, scientifically based field was expected. Applicants must have understood that medicine demanded life-long learning in a rapidly changing, technologically based profession designed to provide care for the suffering. The attitude of the applicant was important and was considered in selection. All academic coursework must have been above average. Applicants were expected to have a GPA of at least 3.0, and if taken, MCAT® scores of 9's and 10's, although no MCAT® score cut-off was utilized. Personal interviews were at the discretion of the Admissions Committee.

GUSM operated under a rolling admissions system although specific deadlines applied to each entering class. Classes started in January, July, and October and students were able to apply to any of these classes.

TUITION AND FINANCIAL AID:

Application Fee: $100 USD (non-refundable)

Payment required to secure acceptance: $1,000 USD (applied to tuition)

Tuition for Basic Sciences: $5,000 USD per module

Tuition for Clinical Sciences: $5,000 USD per module

Graduation Fee: $1,000 USD

Other fees such as laboratory, student, and administrative may have applied.

Grace University was affiliated with Key Resources for the purpose of providing financial aid. The MedAchiever loan, Key Alternative loan, MedAchiever Residency Travel and Relocation loan, and board exam and travel loans were available. United States Federal student loans were not available.

ooooo

Central and South American Medical Schools - Caribbean Region

Hope University School of Medicine

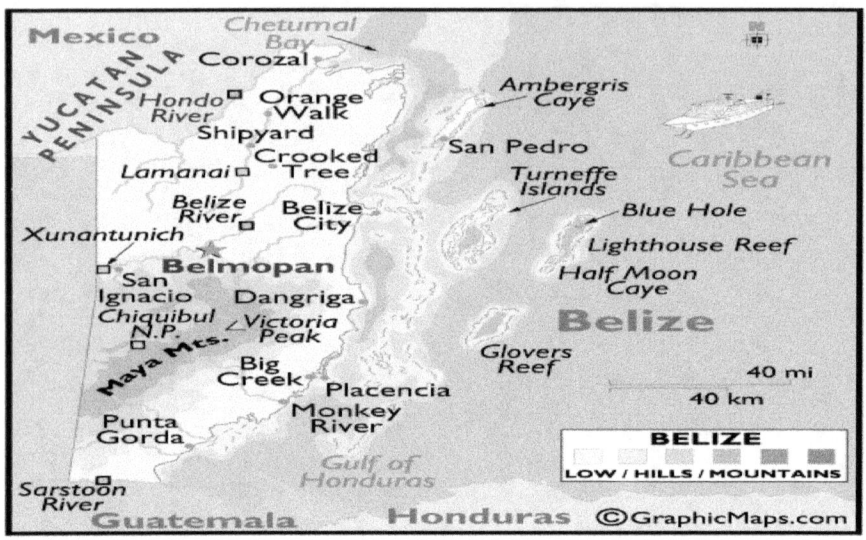

AMRCB® QUICK REFERENCE
Hope University School of Medicine

Years Operated	2005-2007	Currency	BZD
On-Campus Housing	No	Airport Code	BZE
Pre-Medical Program	No	Time Zone	CST (GMT/UTC-6)
MCAT® Required	No	Electricity	110 V
Official Language	English	Driving Side	Right

Hope University School of Medicine

Belize

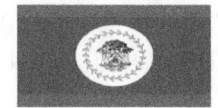

CONTACT INFORMATION:

U.S. Admissions Office
Hope University School of Medicine
7909 Walerga Rd. Suite 112
P.O Box 160
Antelope, California U.S.A. 95843
Telephone: +1 (916) 728-4561
Fax: +1 (888) 235-1076

Campus Address
Hope University School of Medicine
3401 Corner Culvert Road
Belmopan City, Cayo District
Belize

General Information
Website: http://www.hopeuniversity.org/
E-Mail: hopeuniversityinfo@lanset.com

GENERAL INFORMATION:

Hope University School of Medicine was founded in 2005 and operated from 2005 to 2007 in Belmopan, Belize. The school was founded on Christian principles and focused internationally. According to the government in Belize, the charter issued to Hope University School of Medicine was terminated on

September 6th, 2007. The mission of the school was to equip and empower students while emphasizing the holistic approach to health and healing. The University was in cooperation with Hope International Medical Foundation which is a non-profit humanitarian organization.

The school operated with a four-year curriculum that was modeled after the educational system in the United States which was combined with aspects of the European educational system. The MCAT® was not required. The primary campus was in Belmopan Belize with a sub-campus located in Europe in Budapest, Hungary. A combined degree program had begun prior to the school closing as had a two-year Pre-Medical program.

Hope was never certified by the American Medical Residency Certification Board (AMRCB®). Hope was listed by the International Medical Education Directory (IMED), the World Health Organization (WHO), and the Medical Council of Canada (MCC). Hope was chartered and accredited by the Government of Belize. Students were eligible for ECFMG® certification.

CURRICULUM:

Pre-Medical Program

A two year Pre-Medical program was started and was designed to be completed over three semesters. The educational curriculum was designed to highlight the best educational aspects of the European and United States educational systems.

M.D. Program

The curriculum was conducted over a four-year program and could be completed in as little as 40 months. The Basic Sciences were conducted over the first two years followed by two years of clinical training.

Basic Sciences

The Basic Medical Science program was conducted over two years and was offered at the main campus in Belize, Central America and at the sub-campus in Budapest, Hungary

Clinical Sciences

The Clinical clerkships were conducted over the third and fourth years and were available in the United States, Belize, Hungary, the United Kingdom, and other European countries.

Grading

Students were promoted from one semester to the next after passing all courses for that semester and achieved graduation after satisfactorily meeting all performance standards. The Dean promoted a student into the Clinical Science clerkship program only after completing all of the Basic Science program requirements and passing USMLE® Step 1

ENTRANCE REQUIREMENTS:

M.D. Program

The minimum requirement for admission was 90 semester hours of college level courses. Applicants from the United States and Canada were required to have a baccalaureate degree. All applicants were required to complete specific prerequisite coursework, although well qualified applicants could be considered for acceptance after two or three years of college level coursework. International applicants were expected to have completed requirements similar to those in the North American educational system.

The MCAT® was not required.

SELECTION FACTORS:

The Admission Committee selected applicants who possessed intelligence, integrity, and the personal and emotional characteristics necessary to become effective physicians. The Admission Committee based its decision on multiple factors which included the overall undergraduate GPA and overall undergraduate science GPA; the overall graduate GPA if applicable; and the pre-medical GPA. Students were expected to have a strong science background. Letters of recommendations and the personal essay were reviewed. The interview was an important part of the selection process. If applicable, MCAT® scores were reviewed. An applicant's professional, extracurricular, and volunteer experiences were important as well.

TUITION AND FINANCIAL AID:

Tuition for Basic Sciences: $5,500 USD per semester

Tuition for Clinical Sciences: $7,500 USD per semester

Other fees such as laboratory, student, administrative, and graduation may have applied.

Private loans were available. United States Federal student loans were not available.

ooooo

Central and South American Medical Schools - Caribbean Region

InterAmerican Medical University

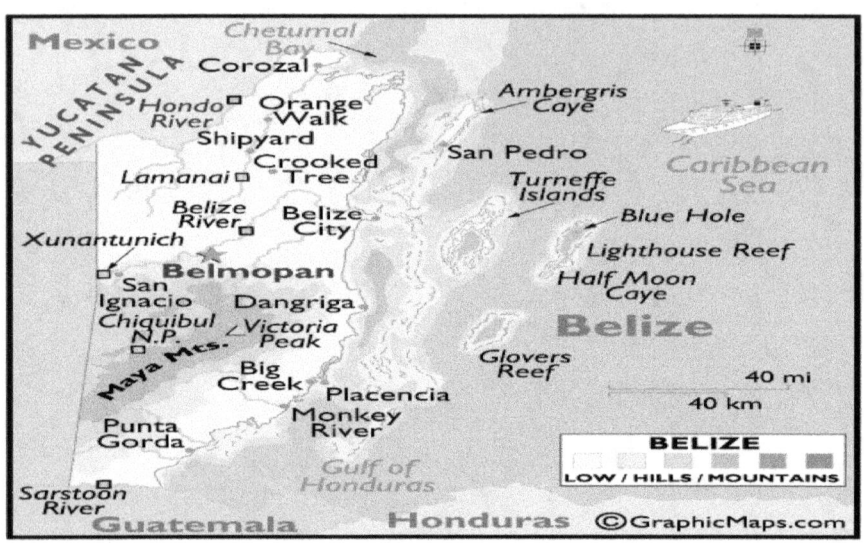

AMRCB® QUICK REFERENCE
InterAmerican Medical University

Years Operated	2003-2006	Currency	BZD
On-Campus Housing	No	Airport Code	BZE
Pre-Medical Program	No	Time Zone	CST (GMT/UTC-6)
MCAT® Required	Yes (North American)	Electricity	110 V
Official Language	English	Driving Side	Right

InterAmerican Medical University

Belize

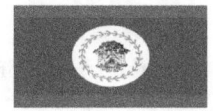

R. Shayne Pavlic, M.I.M. – President
Tiana Pavlic, M.D., M.S.M.E., F.E. – Dean
Romeo A. Pavlic, M.D., M.P.H., M.I.M, M.R.A. – Assistant Dean

CONTACT INFORMATION:

U.S. Admissions Office	Campus Address
InterAmerican Medical University	InterAmerican Medical University
Dean	MM 85.5 Santa Elena Rd.
USA Heart, Inc.	Northern Highway
10 N. Post St., Suite 642	Corozal Town, Corozal District
Spokane, Washington U.S.A. 99201	Belize, Central America
Telephone: (509) 838-0592	Telephone: 011-501-422-3200
Fax: (509) 456-7449	Fax: 011-501-622-6830

General Information
Website: www.interamericanschool.com/
E-Mail: medicine@interamericanschool.com

GENERAL INFORMATION:

InterAmerican Medical University (IMU) was founded 2003 with the first class starting 2003. The school operated under the name of InterAmerican School of Medical Sciences from 2003 through 2006. Small class sizes were utilized. The mission of IMU was to deliver high quality healthcare to Northern Belize.

The curriculum was modeled after the United States system of medical education and operated under the trimester system. A traditional four-year medical curriculum was followed and problem-based learning was utilized. The campus was located on eight acres in with the Bethesda Medical Centre which allowed for early clinical exposure. The campus consisted of a computer lab, student lounge, classrooms, and offices. Additional campus sites were planned for India and Brazil prior to closing.

No on-campus housing was available and students were responsible for arranging their housing, with IMU recommending housings in Corozal Town. On-campus student housing was planned for the future prior to closing. The school operated under a rolling admissions system with classes starting in January, April, and September each year.

IMU was never certified by the American Medical Residency Certification Board (AMRCB®). IMU was listed by the International Medical Education Directory (IMED) and the World Health Organization (WHO). IMU was chartered and accredited by the Government of Belize. Students were eligible for ECFMG® certification.

CURRICULUM:

M.D. Program

The curriculum was conducted over a four-year program consisting of three trimesters each year. The Basic Sciences were conducted over the first six trimesters followed by six clinical trimesters. Patient exposure began early and continued over the first two years in conjunction with the Bethesda Medical Centre.

Basic Sciences

The Basic Sciences were conducted over trimesters one through six on the campus in Corozal Town, Belize.

Central and South American Medical Schools - Caribbean Region

Basic Science Curriculum

Trimester I	Trimester II	Trimester III	Trimester IV	Trimester V	Trimester VI
Medical Interviewing and Presentation	Medical Literature	Epidemiology and Biostatistics	Pathology	Pathology	Pathology
Anatomy and Embryology	Problem Based Learning	Evidence Based Medicine	Pharmacology	Pharmacology	Pharmacology
Biochemistry and Molecular Biology	Biochemistry and Molecular Biology	Genetics	Physiology	Physiology	Physiology
Cell Biology, Physiology, and Histology	Cell Biology, Physiology, and Histology	Immunology	Microbiology	Pathophysiology and Applied Physical Diagnosis	Pathophysiology and Applied Physical Diagnosis
	Physical Diagnosis	Neuroanatomy and Neuroscience	Psychopathology and Pharmacology	Reproduction	Ethics
		Physical Diagnosis	Medicine, Health, and Society		Medical Board Review

Clinical Sciences

The Clinical clerkships were conducted over trimesters seven through twelve and occurred primarily in hospitals in the United States and Belize. Students completed 74 weeks of clinical rotations.

Clinical Science Curriculum

Required – 42 weeks		Selectives – 32 weeks	
Internal Medicine	12 - weeks	Selectives	
Pediatrics	8 - weeks	Neurology	4 - weeks
Surgery	6 - weeks	Intensive Care	4 - weeks
OB/GYN	6 - weeks	Subinternship	4 - weeks
Psychiatry	6 - weeks	Surgical Elective	6 - weeks
Family Medicine	4 - weeks	Ambulatory Medicine	4 – weeks
		Emergency Medicine	4 – weeks
		Electives	
		Student Choice	6 - weeks

Grading

Students were promoted from one semester to the next after passing all courses for that semester and achieved graduation after satisfactorily meeting all performance standards. To be eligible for graduation, all students must have successfully completed all requirements of the curriculum.

ENTRANCE REQUIREMENTS:

M.D. Program

College work must have included the following:

- General Biology or Zoology with labs – one academic year
- Inorganic or General Chemistry with labs – one academic year
- Organic Chemistry with labs – one academic year
- General Physics with labs – one academic course
- Mathematics (Algebra, Pre-Calculus, or Calculus) – one academic course

Courses in Biochemistry and Basic statistics were strongly recommended. Students must have computer and keyboard skills. The MCAT® was required of all North American applicants.

SELECTION FACTORS:

The Admissions Committee reviewed the personal statement of each applicant as well as MCAT® and other comparable test scores. Three letters of recommendation were required as well. The student's entire admission application was reviewed to determine strengths, weaknesses, maturity, motivations for working in the medical field, and overall academic achievements. Applicants were notified within three to five weeks of an admissions decision. All students underwent a background check. There was no application deadline as the school operated under a rolling admissions system with classes starting in January, April, and September.

TUITION AND FINANCIAL AID:

Application Fee: $200 USD (non-refundable)

Matriculation Fee: $1,500 (non-refundable)

Tuition for Basic Sciences (trimesters 1-6): $5,000 USD per trimester

Tuition for Clinical Sciences (trimesters 7-12): $8,000 USD per trimester
Individual Proctor fees applied to some clinical rotations.

Lab Fee: $350 per year

Other fees such as materials, student, administrative, and graduation applied.

United States Federal student loans were not available at this time.

ooooo

Medical University of the Americas

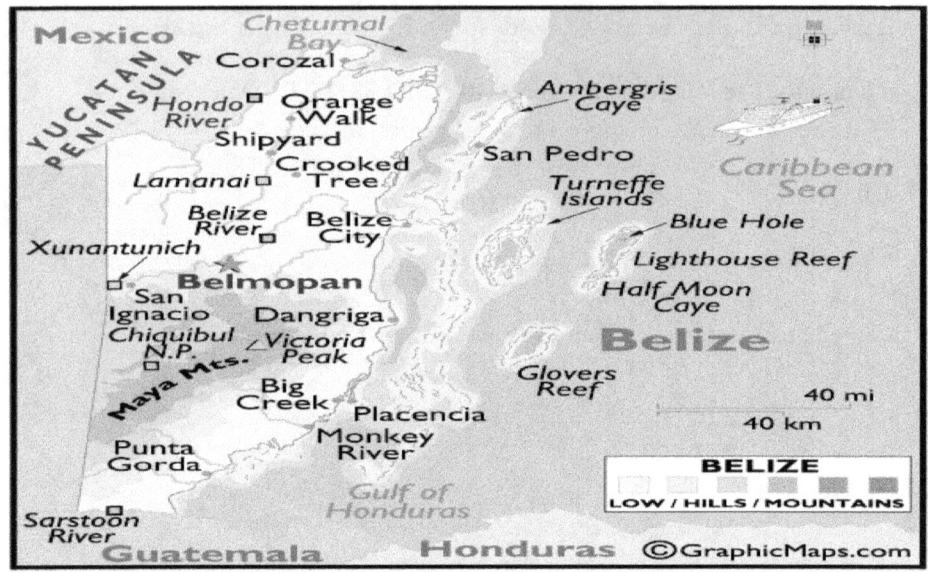

AMRCB® QUICK REFERENCE
Medical University of the Americas

Years Operated	2001-2007	Currency	BZD
On-Campus Housing	No	Airport Code	BZE
Pre-Medical Program	No	Time Zone	CST (GMT/UTC-6)
MCAT® Required	No	Electricity	110 V
Official Language	English	Driving Side	Right

Medical University of the Americas

Belize

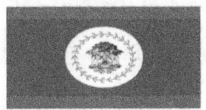

Dr. Jeffrey Sersland - President

CONTACT INFORMATION:

U.S. Admissions Office
Medical University of the Americas
Dean
22 Cross Street
Gardner, Massachusetts 01440 U.S.A.
Telephone: (978) 632-6355

Campus Address
Medical University of the Americas
P.O Box 1271
1000 Coconut Drive
San Pedro Ambergris Caye, Belize
Telephone: (501) 226-3744
Fax (501) 226-3835

General Information
Website: www.mua.edu.bz
E-Mail: muabelize@btl.net

GENERAL INFORMATION:

The Medical University of the Americas – Belize (MUAB) was founded in 2001 and operated from 2001 through 2007. Accreditation was officially terminated by the government of Belize in 2010. MUAB was owned by a parent company,

Medquest, which also owned the Medical University of the Americas. MUAB was associated in the past with the Medical University of the Americas located in Nevis. MUAB sought to "educate tomorrow's doctors" and the curriculum was described as rigorous and designed to prepare students for medical practice in the 21st century.

The campus was located on 7.5 acres and consisted of a main school building. The student/teacher ratio was 6:1. No on-campus student housing existed.

The curriculum was modeled after the United States educational curriculum, operated on a trimester system, and awarded a M.D. degree. The first two years were conducted on the campus in Belize with the clinical rotations taking place abroad. Clinical integration began in the third trimester. The school operated under a rolling admissions system with classes starting in January, May, and September each year.

MUAB was never certified by the American Medical Residency Certification Board (AMRCB®). MUAB was listed by the International Medical Education Directory (IMED) and the World Health Organization (WHO). MUAB was chartered and accredited by the Government of Belize until 2010. Students were eligible for ECFMG® certification.

CURRICULUM:

M.D. Program

The curriculum was conducted over a four-year program. The Basic Sciences were conducted over the first two years followed by two years of clinical rotations. Clinical integration began in the third semester. The curriculum could be completed in as little as 40 months.

Basic Sciences

The Basic Sciences were conducted over five semesters on the campus in Belize.

Clinical Sciences

The Clinical clerkships were conducted over five semesters spanning 72 weeks and occurred in hospitals in the United States as well as other locations.

Grading

In order to graduate, students were required to complete the entire curriculum including five semesters of Basic Sciences and five semesters of the Clinical Science. An overall GPA of 2.0 on a 4-point scale was required in order to be eligible for graduation.

SELECTION FACTORS:

The Admission Committee evaluated each applicant on multiple criteria. Criteria included the overall academic record and intellectual ability, communication skills, and goals for entering the medical field. Letters of recommendation were reviewed and the Admission Committee sought to understand the special interests, hobbies, and talents of each applicant. International travel and knowledge of international education were beneficial. Students were sought who could function in a team, respond to stress, display flexibility, and accept responsibility. The Admissions Committee sought to identify personal qualities such as motivation, judgment, enthusiasm, and spontaneity. Students were scheduled for an interview within two weeks of receipt of all application documents. Personal interviews and conference calls were both utilized for the interview process. Applicants were notified within 10 days of an admissions decision. The school operated under a rolling admissions system with classes starting in January, May, and September each year.

TUITION AND FINANCIAL AID:

Application Fee: $75 USD (non-refundable)

Tuition for Basic Sciences (semester 1-5): $5,500 USD per semester

Tuition for Clinical Sciences (semester 6-10): $7,900 USD per semester

Other fees such as laboratory, student, administrative, and graduation may have applied.

United States Federal student loans were not available.

ooooo

Central and South American Medical Schools - Caribbean Region

St. Luke's University School of Medicine

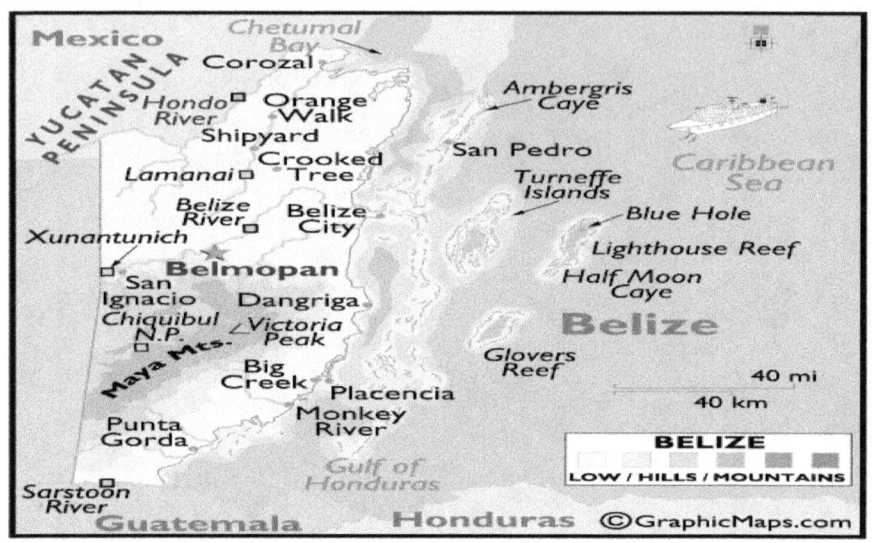

AMRCB® QUICK REFERENCE
St. Luke's University School of Medicine

Years Operating	2002-2007	Currency	BZD
On-Campus Housing	No	Airport Code	BZE
Pre-Medical Program	No	Time Zone	CST (GMT/UTC-6)
MCAT® Required	No	Electricity	110 V
Official Language	English	Driving Side	Right

St. Luke's University School of Medicine

Belize

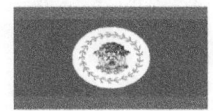

Dr. Shrinivas Murthy – Academic Dean

CONTACT INFORMATION:

Prior Campus Address
St. Luke's University School of Medicine
P.O Box 557
Belmopan, Cayo Belize
Telephone: (877) 545-8537
Fax: 011-501-822-1252

Prior Campus Address
St. Luke's University SOM
P.O. Box 1773
Belize City, Belize
Telephone: (501) 822-1250

Prior Campus Address
St. Luke's University SOM
P.O. Box 240
Barrier Reef Drive
San Pedro Town, Ambergris Caye, Belize
Telephone: 011-501-226-2912

General Information
Website: www.stluke.edu.bz
E-Mail: admissions@stluke.edu.bz
Telephone: (877) 540-LUKES (in U.S.)

GENERAL INFORMATION:

St. Luke's University School of Medicine was founded in 2002 and operated from 2202 – 2007. Operations officially ceased in October of 2007. It is noted that several complaints from students were recorded against the school. In addition to the campus in Belize, campuses in Monrovia, Liberia and Cape Coast, Ghana were both listed as well, but it is unclear if any education actually took place at any location other than in Belize. Approximately 75 students were educated at the University.

The medical school curriculum was modeled after the educational system in the United States and a Doctor of Medicine and Surgery degree was granted. The Guiding Principles of St. Luke's was to prepare physicians in the 21st century for practice using wisdom of the past while utilizing technology, and while not losing sight of the human element of medicine. The stated desire was to form effective diagnosticians that could balance hard science and heartfelt sensitivity. Small class sizes were utilized with hands-on clinical training starting in the first two years. No on-campus student housing options were available.

St. Luke's was never certified by the American Medical Residency Certification Board (AMRCB®). St. Luke's was listed by the International Medical Education Directory (IMED) and the World Health Organization (WHO). St. Luke's was chartered and accredited by the Government of Belize. Initial publications reported accreditation in the Republic of Liberia and the Republic of Ghana in West Africa, but this was not able to be confirmed and was in question. Students were eligible for ECFMG® certification.

CURRICULUM:

M.D. Program

The curriculum was conducted over a four-year program. Clinical training began in the first two years of Basic Science education. The Clinical clerkships were reported as being conducted in the United States.

ENTRANCE REQUIREMENTS:

M.D. Program

The MCAT® was not required.

TUITION AND FINANCIAL AID:

Tuition for Basic Sciences: $8,775 USD per semester

Tuition for Clinical Sciences: $9,875 USD per semester

Other fees such as laboratory, student, administrative, and graduation may have applied.

Private loans were available from outside sources. United States Federal student loans were not available.

ooooo

St. Matthew's University School of Medicine – (Cayman Islands)

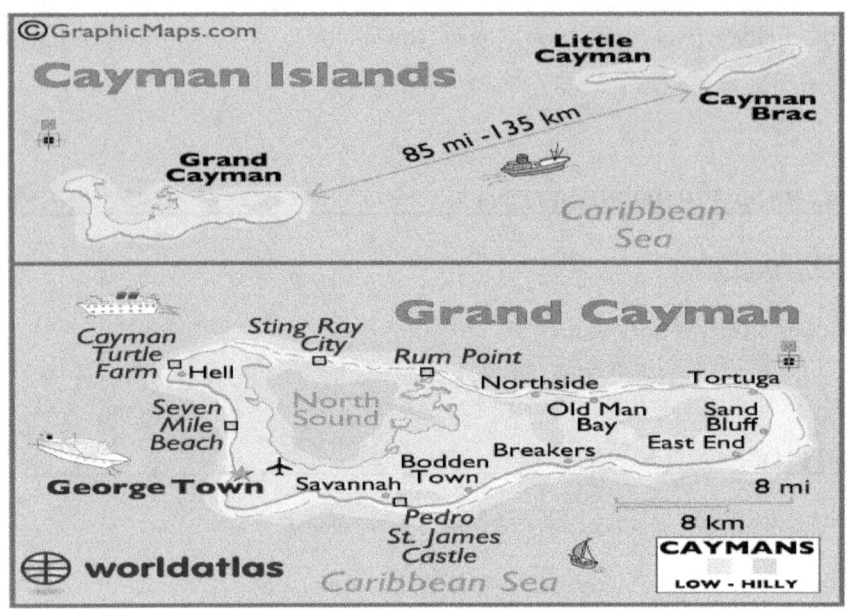

AMRCB® QUICK REFERENCE
St. Matthew's University School of Medicine

Year Founded	1997	**Currency**	KYD
On-Campus Housing	Yes	**Airport Code**	GCM
Pre-Medical Program	No	**Time Zone**	EST (GMT/UTC-5)
MCAT® Required	Yes (U.S. citizens only)	**Electricity**	110 V
Official Language	English	**Driving Side**	Left

St. Matthew's University School of Medicine

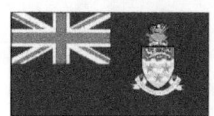

CONTACT INFORMATION:

U.S. Admission Office
U. S. Administrative Offices
St. Matthew's University
12124 High Tech Avenue
Suite 350
Orlando, Florida 32817 U.S.A.

Campus Address
St. Matthews's University
Lime Tree Bay Ave
West Bay, Cayman Islands

General Information
Telephone: 1-800-498-9700 or 407-977-8100
Fax: 1-800-565-7177
Website: http://www.stmatthews.edu/
E-Mail: admissions@stmatthews.edu

GENERAL INFORMATION:

St. Matthew's University School of Medicine was founded in 1997 and operated in the country of Belize until 2002. In 2002, St. Matthew's University School of Medicine permanently moved the medical school campus to the Cayman Islands in the Caribbean and is currently in full operation in this location. The complete medical school entry for St. Matthew's University School of Medicine can be found on page 159 of the AMRCB® publication entitled: Caribbean Medical Schools Based on a U.S. Curriculum – Greater and Lesser Antilles. Forty additional medical schools in the Caribbean region, which are not included in this current publication, are described in that publication.

○○○○○

Washington University of Health and Sciences

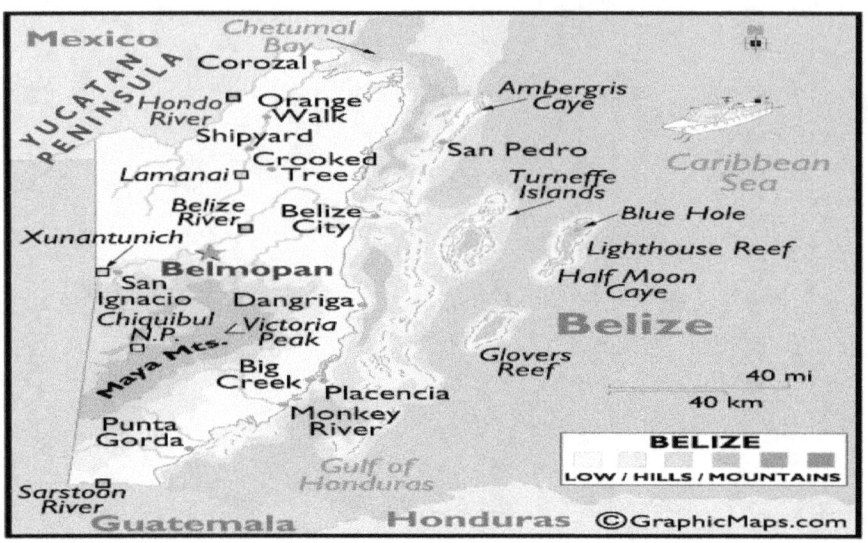

AMRCB® QUICK REFERENCE
Washington University of Health and Sciences

Year Founded	2012	Currency	BZD
On-Campus Housing	Yes	Airport Code	BZE
Pre-Medical Program	Yes	Time Zone	CST (GMT/UTC-6)
MCAT® Required	No	Electricity	110 V
Official Language	English	Driving Side	Right

Washington University of Health and Sciences

Belize

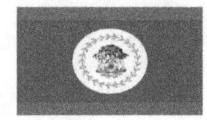

Dr. Malik J. Soudah – President and CEO
Robert T. Fredrick, M.D. – Executive Dean

CONTACT INFORMATION:

U.S. Admissions Office
Washington University of
Health Sciences
c/o American Academic Services
2602 Oakstone Dr. Suite 6
Columbus, Ohio U.S.A. 43231
Telephone: (866) 966-9843
Fax: (614) 340-4688

Campus Address
Washington University of
Health Sciences
Seagrape Drive
San Pedro, Ambergris Caye
Belize
Telephone: 011-1-501-226-2682

General Information
Website: http://www.wuhs.org/
E-Mail: admssions@wuhs.org

GENERAL INFORMATION:

The Washington University of Health Sciences (WUHS) was initially founded in 2012 with classes starting in 2012. WUHS bases the educational model on effective communications; basic clinical skills; lifelong learning; self-awareness; social and community context; and developing the skills to guide diagnosis, management, therapeutics, and prevention. The mission of the school is to support a community of professionals committed to excellence in the education of highly qualified students in medicine. The core values of WUHS are integrity, respect, honesty, and professionalism. Class sizes are small to allow for a low student / teacher ratio.

The curriculum is modeled after United States medical schools and follows a problem-based curriculum. The curriculum is a competency based curriculum that balances excellent clinical training with strong interpersonal and professional skills. WUHS utilizes a state of the art pathway to design the educational model for the individual student learning style. A Pre-Medical program is available for students who have not yet completed the required prerequisites.

The campus has modern classrooms and laboratory facilities. WUHS has an investment plan which includes infrastructure and technology platforms. On and off-campus housing is currently available and fees vary depending upon occupancy and amenities. Current housing costs range from $300-700 USD per semester. No admissions deadline is in place as the school operates under a rolling admissions system with classes starting in January, May, and September.

WUHS is not currently certified by the American Medical Residency Certification Board (AMRCB®). WUHS is listed by the International Medical Education Directory (IMED) and the World Health Organization (WHO). WUHS is chartered and accredited by the Government of Belize. Students are eligible for ECFMG® certification.

CURRICULUM:

Pre-Medical Program

The pre-medical program is conducted over one year spanning three semesters. The instruction takes place on the WUHS campus in Belize. Upon completion, students can directly apply to the M.D. program.

Pre-Medical Curriculum

Pre-Med Semester I	Pre-Med Semester II	Pre-Med Semester III
General Biology I	College Physics I	General Biology II
General Chemistry I	General Chemistry II	Organic Chemistry II
Algebra I	Organic Chemistry I	College Physics II
Medical English Literature, Writing, and Oral Expression I	Medical English Literature, Writing, and Oral Expression II	

M.D. Program

The curriculum is conducted over a four-year program spanning 11 semesters. WUHS utilizes a problem-based curriculum as well as case studies and small group discussion. The integrated pathway consists of organ system education. The Basic Sciences are conducted over the first five semesters, with a fifth "bridge" semester in place which transitions students into the five Clinical Science rotations. Patient exposure begins early from the second week of classes at supervised local clinics.

Basic Sciences

The Basic Sciences are conducted over five 15-week semesters on the campus in San Pedro, Belize. The fifth semester includes an integrated USMLE® course and an Introduction to Clinical Medicine course that takes place in a U.S. hospital in either Florida or Chicago.

Basic Science Curriculum

Semester I	Semester II	Semester III	Semester IV	Semester V
Gross and Developmental Anatomy with lab	Behavioral Science	Microbiology	Systemic Pathology II with lab	Intro to Clinical Medicine
Histology and Cell Biology with lab	Physiology with lab	Immunology	Pharmacology with lab	Physical Diagnosis
Embryology lab	Neuroscience / Neuro-Anatomy	General Pathology I with lab	Legal and Medical Ethics	USMLE® Review
Biochemistry with lab	Medical Nutrition	Medical Genetics	USMLE® Grand Rounds	
Medical Terminology	USMLE® Grand Rounds	Epidemiology / Biostatistics		
USMLE® Grand Rounds		USMLE® Grand Rounds		

Clinical Sciences

The Clinical clerkships are conducted over semesters six through eleven spanning 72 weeks and occur in hospitals in the United States and United Kingdom.

Rotations in Europe and Asia may be available as well. WUHS has major clinical hubs in the United States in Denver, Colorado and Chicago, Illinois.

Clinical Science Curriculum

Required – 48 weeks		Electives and Selectives – 30 weeks	
General Medicine	8 - weeks	Selectives	
Surgery	8 - weeks	Seriously Ill Hospitalized Patients	4 - weeks
Pediatrics	8 - weeks	Emergency Medicine	4 - weeks
OB/GYN	6 - weeks	Ambulatory Care in Internal Medicine	4 - weeks
Psychiatry	4 - weeks	Chronic care	4 - weeks
Family Medicine	4 - weeks	Electives	
Neurology	4 - weeks	Electives	14 - weeks
Common Invasive Procedures and Elective	6 - weeks		

Grading

Students are promoted from one semester to the next after passing all courses for that semester and achieve graduation after satisfactorily meeting all performance standards. The Dean promotes a student into the Clinical Science clerkship program only after completing all of the Basic Science program requirements and passing USMLE® Step 1.

ENTRANCE REQUIREMENTS:

Pre-Medical Program

The program is available for students who have not yet completed the necessary prerequisites to gain admission into WUHS. Applicants are expected to have a successful academic background.

M.D. Program

The minimum requirement for admission is 90 semester hours of college level courses. A baccalaureate degree or equivalent is highly recommended. A minimum GPA of 2.75 is required. College work must include the following (Lab work is nearly universally expected even when not listed):

- General Biology or Zoology – one academic year
- Inorganic or General Chemistry – one academic year
- Organic Chemistry – one academic year
- General Physics – one academic year
- English – three academic classes

- College Mathematics – two academic courses

Courses in sociology, political sciences, psychology, anthropology, and economics are recommended. The MCAT® is optional and submitted scores should have been taken within the last two years. Applicants are strongly urged to take the MCAT®.

SELECTION FACTORS:

WUHS strives to select students who have demonstrated excellence, integrity, respect, professionalism, and that fit with the core values and guiding principles of the institution. Students are sought who have demonstrated excellence in education, research, and patient care. Prospective applicants are expected to embrace the highest standards of ethical behaviors and moral character. The Admission Committee strives to select applicants while keeping in sight the ethical principles, human values, and spiritual dimensions necessary to practice medicine. The MCAT® is optional but strongly recommended. Students are urged to take the course in the spring prior to applying for medical school. Students are required to have a letter of recommendation from the Pre-Medical Committee of the undergraduate institution attended as well as two letters of recommendation from science professors. The Admissions Committee considers the personal traits, academic qualifications, and results of the MCAT® in the selection process. The Admissions Committee seeks to identify students who will succeed in the medical education. The personal statement and personal interviews are important in the selection process as well. There is no application deadline as the school operates under a rolling admissions system with classes starting in January, May, and September.

TUITION AND FINANCIAL AID:

Application Fee: $100 USD (non-refundable)

Enrollment reservation fee: $1,000 USD (non-refundable)

Reservation Fee: $500 USD (one-time)

Tuition for Pre-Medical Sciences (semester 1-3): $4,900 USD per semester

Tuition for Basic Sciences (semester 1-5): $5,900 USD per semester

Tuition for Clinical Sciences (semester 6-11): $7,600 USD per semester

Graduation Fee: $1200 USD for final graduation. $250 USD each for Premed and Basic Science graduation.

USMLE® Step 2 Fee: $500 USD

Other fees such as laboratory, student, and administrative may apply.

Scholarships and payment options are available based on academic performance, need, and profession and professional background. United States Federal student loans are not available at this time.

ooooo

BELIZE INFORMATION

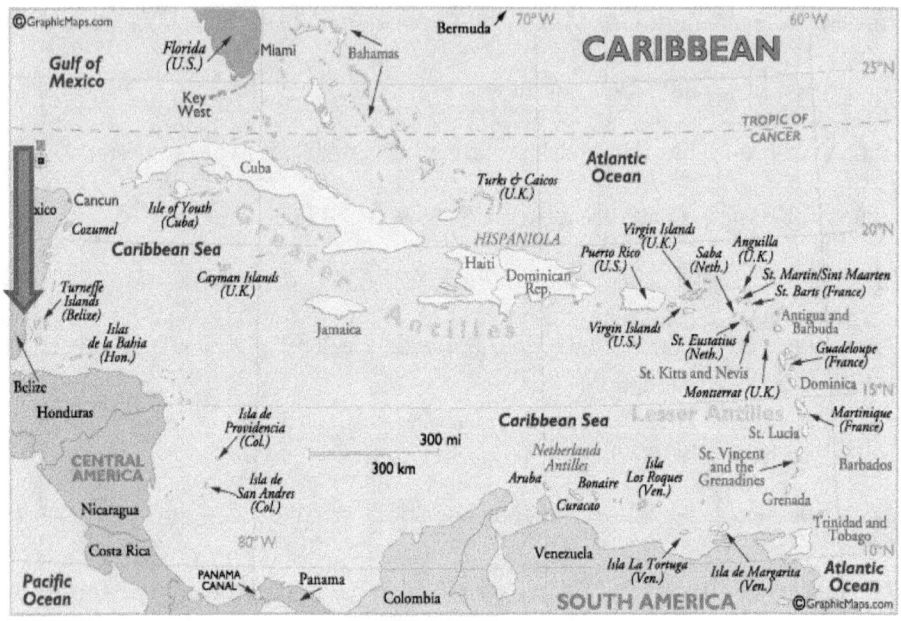

Belize is located on the Northeastern coast of Central America and has an area of 8,867 square miles (22,966 km²). The country is bordered by the Caribbean Sea on the East, Guatemala on the West and South, and Mexico on the North. The highest point is Doyle's Delight at 3,687 feet (1124m). The second largest barrier reef in the world at 185 miles (298 km) is located offshore. Over 40% of the country is protected as parks and reserves. The population density is low for Central America with a total population of just over 330,000 persons. The capital city is Belmopan city with a population 14,500 persons. The American Global campus is located in Ladyville in Belize City as is the campuses of CAHSU. St. Luke's campus was located in Belize City as well while in operation. The

InterAmerican campus was located in Corozal Town while in operation. The campus of Avicina is located in Belmopan City and the campuses of Grace and Hope were in Belmopan City while in operation. Washington University is in San Pedros Ambergris Caye and the Medical University of the Americas was located there as well while in operation.

Belize gained independence from Britain in 1981 and is an independent nation within the British Commonwealth. Belize is officially a unitary parliamentary constitutional monarchy and has a democratically elected government. The Queen of England is the head of state and she is represented by the Governor General of Belize. The Prime Minister is the head of government. Belize had been known previously as British Honduras from 1862 to 1973. Belize is a member of the CARICOM organization.

The culture is influenced heavily by Mayan and Spanish influences. Many religious denominations are represented and include Anglican, Baptist, Jehovah Witnesses, Methodist, Roman Catholic, and Seventh Day Adventist. The population consists of 25% Belize Creole, 8% Caucasian, 64% Mexican/Mayan/local indigenous tribes, with the rest of the population made up of small numbers of other international groups. The official language is English although an English based Creole is often spoken as well as Spanish and Mayan. Belize is the only country in the region where English is the official language.

The climate ranges from tropical to subtropical depending on geography. The average temperature is 80°F (27°C) year round. The seasons of the year are marked primarily by changes of humidity instead of changes in temperature. The country has a wet season from June to November and a dry season from December to May. Yearly average rainfall ranges from 53 inches (1350 mm) in the North to 177 inches (4,500 mm) in the South. Hurricane season runs from June through November and the country has been impacted several by hurricane throughout its history.

The economy consists of farming, petroleum production, sugar cane processing, fishing, and tourism. Drug trafficking has been an issue in Belize. The official currency is the Belize dollar (BZD) with an exchange rate of two BZD to one USD. The national tax is 12.5% on all goods and services. The time zone is UTC-6 which is the same as the Central Standard Time Zone in the United States. Electricity is 110 volts which is the same as in North America.

The main airport is the Philip S. W. Goldson International Airport (BZE) located in Belize City. The airport is currently undergoing expansion and is the busiest airport in the country and is a 30 minute drive from Belize City's center in Ladyville. International flights are available from major U.S. destinations including Atlanta, GA; Dallas, TX; Charlotte, NC; and Miami, Florida. Major airlines servicing Belize include American Airlines, Continental airlines, Delta Air lines, U.S. Airways, and Brupo TACA. Several local airlines are available as well which connect Belize to Guatemala and Mexico. Driving is on the right hand side just as in North America. Car travel from Mexico and Central America is an alternative way to access the country as well and Belize has four major highways. Water ferries are an option from regional cities as well

ooooo

Central and South American Medical Schools - Caribbean Region

Columbus University School of Medicine and Health Sciences

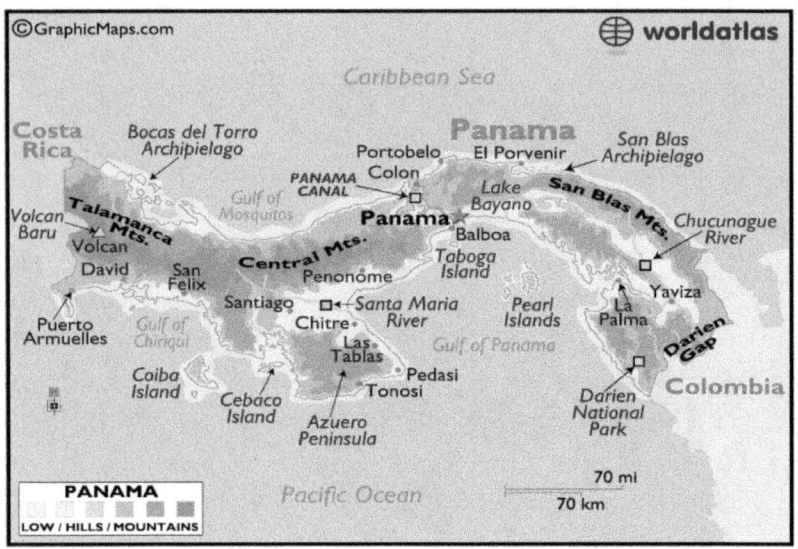

AMRCB® QUICK REFERENCE			
Columbus University School of Medicine and Health Sciences			
Year Founded	1992	Currency	PAB
On-Campus Housing	No	Airport Code	PTY
Pre-Medical Program	Yes	Time Zone	EST (GMT/UTC-5)
MCAT® Required	No	Electricity	110 V
Official Language	Spanish	Driving Side	Right

Columbus University School of Medicine and Health Sciences

Panama

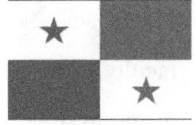

Dr. Prabhaker Tummala – CEO College of Medicine
Dr. Carlos Arellann Lenox – Principle
Dr. Luis Garrido, M.D. – Vice Dean of Academics
Dr. Robert Samuels Halphen – Director of Student Affairs College of Medicine

CONTACT INFORMATION:

U.S. Admissions Office
Columbus University College of
Medicine and Health Sciences
6956 East Broad Street
Suite 400
Columbus, Ohio 43213 U.S.A.
Telephone: (909) 945-7687
Fax: +507 263-3896

Campus Address
Columbus University College of
Medicine and Health Sciences
Edificio Vigamar I
Avenica Justo Arosemena y Calle 39
Panama
Telephone: (507) 263-3892 -or-
263-3888 204-1400

General Information
Website: http://2nsc-2010-a.com/
E-Mail: Columbus@columbus.edu

GENERAL INFORMATION:

The Columbus University College of Medicine and Health Sciences (COMHS) was founded in 1992 with the first medical school class starting in 1996. COMHS strives to solve the shortage of well-trained physician's world-wide while providing a personalized education to students. The school seeks to train students in all disciplines of medicine. Over 350 students have graduated from the school since classes began and the school accepts approximately 100 students per year. The typical student/faculty ration is 50:1. COMHS strives to attract students from the international community.

The medical curriculum takes place over 6 years and is taught in English and Spanish. The curriculum starts with 2 semesters of a Pre-Medical Track. The curriculum is designed to produce medical professionals with excellent clinical, rehabilitative, therapeutic, and preventive skills. An International track is also available where students spend their first year in Panama and subsequent years at other locations. Additional Schools in the system include Administrative Sciences; Economics and Business; Education and Linguistics; Marine Sciences and Technology; Natural Sciences and Technology; Social Sciences; Information Technology; and Law and Political Science. The school does help with residency placement for outstanding students upon graduation.

COMHS has two main campuses. The main campus is located in Panama City, Panama, and the second campus is located in David, Panama. Both campuses are fully equipped and offer a fully functioning laboratory, state-of-the-art medical equipment and training devices, and classrooms. Columbus University currently has an affiliation with the University of Texas Medical School at Houston. No on-campus housing is currently available with off-campus housing costs ranging from $500-700 USD per month.

COMHS is not currently certified by the American Medical Residency Certification Board (AMRCB®). COMHS is listed by the International Medical Education Directory (IMED) and the World Health Organization (WHO). COMHS is ISO 9001-2000 Certified. COMHS is chartered and accredited by the Panamanian Ministry of Education. Students are eligible for ECFMG® certification.

CURRICULUM:

Pre-Medical Program

The curriculum starts with the pre-medical curriculum spanning the first two semesters.

Pre-Medical Curriculum

Semester I	Semester II
Methods of Study	Molecular and Cellular Biology
General Administration	Ecology and the Environment
General Biology	Organic Chemistry
Mathematics	Physical Chemistry
General Psychology	English II
Inorganic Chemistry	Spanish
English I	Intro to Sociology
History of Panama	Geography of Panama

M.D. Program

The curriculum is conducted over 10 semesters spanning five years. Instruction takes place in classrooms, blended learning systems, and via distance or virtual education systems. The use of technology is expanded in the curriculum

Basic Sciences

The Basic Sciences are conducted over four semesters on either of the campuses in Panama. Semesters span 15 weeks in length. A USMLE® review course takes place between the Basic Sciences and Clinical Sciences.

Basic Science Curriculum

Semester III	Semester IV	Semester V	Semester VI
Anatomy	Immunology	Physiology	Genetics
Embryology	Microbiology	Pharmacology	Nutrition
Histology	Parasitology	Introduction to Medical Practice	Philosophy and the History of Medicine
English	Neuroanatomy	First Aid and CPR	Public Health
Biochemistry	Medical Information	Medical Sociology	Anatomical Pathology
		Medical Anthropology	Clinical Pathophysiology
		Biostatistics and Demographics	Medical Psychology

Clinical Sciences

The Clinical clerkships are conducted over six semesters and occur in Panama, the United Kingdom, and in the United States. Teaching takes place at Hospital Santo Tomás which is the largest Public hospital in Panama.

Clinical Science Curriculum

Semester VII	Semester VIII	Semester IX
Diagnostic Radiology	Dermatology	Family Medicine
Community Medicine I	Community Medicine II	Orthopedics
Epidemiology Clinic	Legal Medicine	Psychiatry/Behavioral Sciences
Psychopathology	Pediatrics I	Pediatrics II
Internal Medicine I	Internal Medicine II	Obstetrics
Occupational Medicine	Electrocardiograms	Ophthalmology
Hematology	Accounting for Physicians	Otolaryngology
Semester X	**Semester XI**	**Semester XII**
Surgery	Geriatrics	Practice of Externship
Urology	Urgent Care	Internal Medicine
Gynecology	Neurology	Surgery
Internal Medicine III	Therapeutics	Pediatrics
Dermatology	Correlative Imaging	OB/GYN
Clinical Toxicology	Surgery II	
Preventive Medicine	Health Service Administration	

Grading

Students are promoted from one semester to the next after passing all courses for that semester and achieve graduation after satisfactorily meeting all performance standards. The Dean promotes a student into the Clinical Science clerkship program only after completing all of the Basic Science program requirements. Students must maintain good moral practices within and outside of the university. Students must be fluent in a second language (Spanish, French, or English) in order to graduate.

ENTRANCE REQUIREMENTS:

National Students

Students from Panama must have obtained and submit proof of the following:

- A Bachelor of Science degree
- Secondary studies credits
- Two Copies of a reference of conduct
- Two copies of the certificate of personal identity
- Two passport-sized photos
- Certificate of good physical and mental health.

Foreign Students

- Bachelor of Science degree registered and authenticated by the Ministry of Foreign Affairs of the country of origin and authenticated by the Consulate of Panama
- Secondary studies credits registered and authenticated by the Ministry of Foreign Affairs of the country of origin and authenticated by the Consulate of Panama
- Two copies of reference of conduct
- Two passport-size photographs
- Certificate of good physical and mental health
- Compulsory preparatory course

SELECTION FACTORS:

Transfer students are considered. COMHS seeks dedicated students and no specific majors are preferred. Students are not required to take the MCAT®. A GPA of 3.0 or higher is required in order to be eligible for selection at COMHS. Applicants are able to defer acceptance on a case-by-case basis. A science major is not required for selection although all science prerequisites must have been completed. COMHS selects students that exhibit values of the institution. Recognized values include: excellence and academic quality; responsibility; commitment; honesty; loyalty; efficiency; cooperation; teamwork; leadership; and creativity.

TUITION AND FINANCIAL AID:

Application Fee: none

Registration Fee: $500 USD (one-time fee)

Enrollment Reservation Fee: $1,000 USD

Tuition for Pre-Medical Sciences: $4,900 per semester

Tuition for Basic Sciences: $5,900 USD per semester

Tuition for Clinical Sciences: $7,600 USD per semester

USMLE® Review (5th semester): $1,850 USD

VISA Processing Fee: $200 USD

Graduation Fee: $1,000 USD.

Other fees such as laboratory, student government, and administrative may apply.

Several scholarships including merit based and geographic are available. Private loans may be available from outside sources. United States Federal student loans are not available at this time.

ooooo

Central and South American Medical Schools - Caribbean Region

Central and South American Medical Schools - Caribbean Region

PANAMA INFORMATION

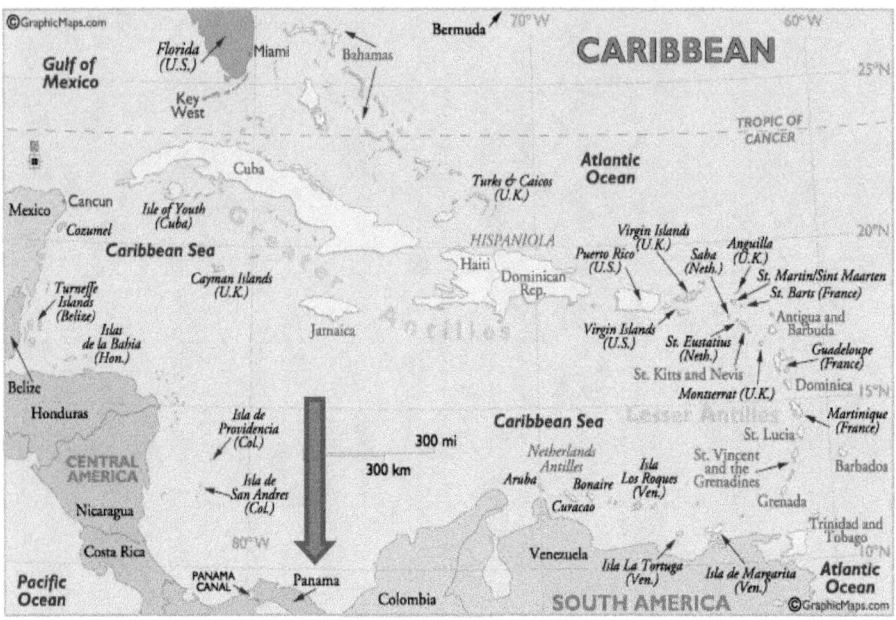

Panama is located on the isthmus that connects North and South America. Panama is bordered by the Caribbean on the North, the Pacific Ocean on the South, Costa Rica on the west, and Columbia to the southwest. Panama has an area of 46,922 square miles (75,515 km²) and is the southernmost country in Central America and all of North America. The highest point is Volcan Baru at 11,401 feet (3,475m). The population of panama is 3.6 million with a population density of 140.6 persons per square mile. The capital and largest city is Panama City and over half of the population of the country lives in the capital city or the surrounding metro area. The Columbus University School of Medicine and

Health Sciences has campuses located in the Panama City as well as in David, Panama which is located 5 hours by car to the west of Panama City.

Panama is officially called the Republic of Panama and gained independence from Spain in 1821 after nearly 300 years of Spanish rule. Panama was then considered a department of Columbia for the next eighty years and eventually gained independence once more in 1903 with the backing of the United States. Panama was invaded by the United States in 1989 in an effort to stabilize the country and to protect civilian lives based on years of corruption. Significant stabilization of the country occurred after several political regime changes by the early 21st century. Construction of the Panama Canal began in 1904 and ownership for the canal was transferred from the United States back to Panama in 1999. Panama was initially settled by the Spanish in the 16th century and was inhabited by different indigenous tribes prior to this. Panama is officially a unitary presidential constitutional republic although it was a constitutional democracy dominated by a commercially oriented oligarchy from 1903 through 1968

The culture is influenced heavily by Mesito, Caribbean, and Spanish influences. Ethnic groups in Panama consist of 70% Mesito, 14% Zambo, 10% Caucasian, and 6% Amerindian. Over 75% of the country identifies as Roman Catholic, 20% as Christian, with several other faiths represented in small numbers including Jehovah Witnesses, Methodist, Jewish, and Seventh Day Adventist. The official language is Spanish and this is the first language of 93% of the population although many citizens speak both Spanish and English.

The climate of Panama is tropical. Temperatures are high throughout the country with minimal seasonal variation and range from 75-90°F (24-30°C) year round. Temperatures are cooler in the mountains and on the Pacific side in comparison with the Caribbean side. The country has a wet season from April to December but this can vary by seven to nine months each year. Yearly average rainfall ranges from 51 inches (1295 mm) on the Pacific side to 118 inches (2997 mm) on the Caribbean side. Panama has only been impacted by one hurricane in 1969 since records have been kept.

The economy of Panama is significantly supported by tolls from the Panama Canal and is the second largest economy in Central America. The economy also is supported by banking, tourism, commerce, and trading. Recently retirement from foreign citizens and real estate has become important contributors to the economy. The current unemployment rate is 2.7%. The official currency is the Panamanian Balboa (PAB) with an exchange rate of 1.0 PAB to 1.0 USD. U.S. dollars are used as paper currency in the country although Panama issues its own coinage. The time zone is UTC-5 which is the same as the Eastern Standard Time Zone in the United States. Electricity is 110 volts which is the same as in North America although some regional variations may be found through the county.

The main airport is the Tocumen International Airport (PTY) located 15 miles from Panama City and this is the largest airport in Central America. The airport underwent renovations in 2006 and is the busiest airport in Central America as well. It serves as a regional hub for Central and South America as well as the Caribbean. International flights are available from major U.S. destinations, Canada, and Europe. Driving is on the right hand side just as in North America.

ooooo

Aureus University School of Medicine

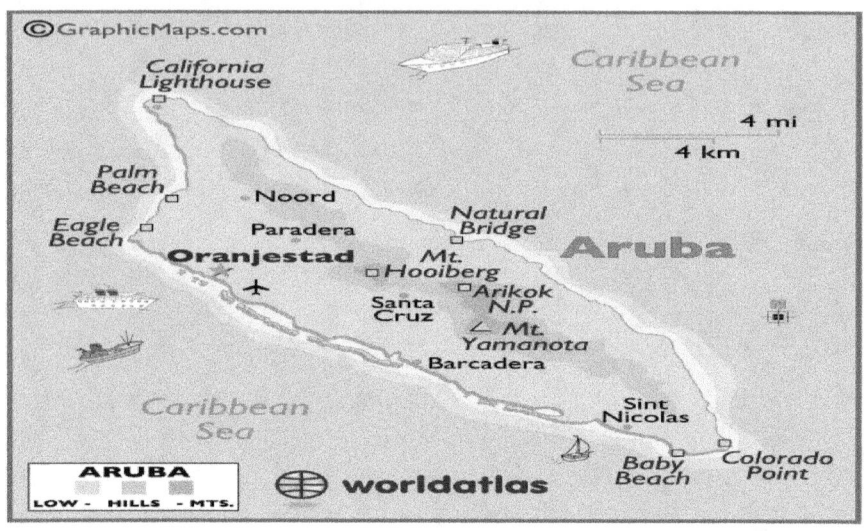

AMRCB® QUICK REFERENCE
Aureus University School of Medicine

Year Founded	2004	Currency	AWG
On-Campus Housing	Yes	Airport Code	AUA
Pre-Medical Program	Yes	Time Zone	EST (GMT/UST-5)
MCAT® Required	No	Electricity	110 V
Official Language	Dutch	Driving Side	Right

Aureus University School of Medicine

Aruba

Gurmit Chilana, M.D. - Executive Dean
Theodore P. Gluedk - Chief Operating Officer
Mukhtar Nandra, M.D. - Director of Clinical Affairs

CONTACT INFORMATION:

U.S. Admission Office
21-00 Route 208 South, Suite 220
Fair Lawn, New Jersey 07410 U.S.A.

Campus Address
Wayaca 31C
Oranjestad, Aruba

General Information
Telephone: 866-596-9919 or 297-583-2126
Fax: 297-583-2127
Website: http://www.aureusuniversity.com
E-Mail: via contact form at: http://www.aureusuniversity.com/contact-us/

GENERAL INFORMATION:

Aureus University School of Medicine (AUSM) was established in 2004. AUSM was formally known as the All Saints University of Medicine. AUSM desires to prepare medical students to become exemplary, efficient, and ethical physicians. The mission of the school is to provide students with the solid foundation in medicine needed to overcome challenges in their medical careers while providing an affordable, first-rate medical education. The motto of AUSM is MEDICAE MANUS which means "healing hands to the four corners of the globe."

AUSM has plans in place to expand the campus including research and fitness facilities, laboratories, and to fully equip the campus with state-of-the-art equipment. Over 20,000 square feet (1860 m²) of educational space will be available as well as a modern cafeteria and gymnasium. On-campus student housing became available in 2012, and students may choose to live on or off campus at this time. Campus housing preference is given to new students and is currently $300-$450 monthly depending on occupancy.

The curriculum is modeled after the North American educational system. A pre-medical program is available and offered exclusively at Canadian locations for three years followed by clinical rotations in the United States. AUSM now has a pilot program in place that currently allows select students to complete their Basic Sciences in Brampton, Ontario or Surrey, British Columbia instead of the Aruba campus. Transfer students may be admitted depending on individual credentials and can transfer into the Clinical Science rotations and must pass the Clinical Basic Science Exam (CBSE). There is no admissions deadline in place as the school operates under a rolling admissions system with starting classes in January, May, and September.

AUSM is listed by the International Medical Education Directory (IMED), the World Health Organization (WHO), and is listed with the Medical Council of Canada (MCC). Students are eligible for ECFMG® certification. AUSM is not currently certified by the American Medical Residency Certification Board (AMRCB®).

CURICULUM:

Pre-Medical Program (5 Year MD Program)

This program is conducted on the Aruba campus; in Brampton, Ontario; or Surrey, British Columbia and is conducted over three semesters that are each 16 weeks long. The curriculum involves three semesters which allow for the completion of the pre-medical requirements. Coursework includes Biology, Chemistry, Physics, English, and Mathematics. Upon successful completion, students will begin the Basic Sciences.

Pre-Medical Curriculum

Semester I	Semester II	Semester III
Biology	Mathematics	Medical Terminology
General Chemistry	Organic Chemistry	Introductory Anatomy
Physics	English	Introductory Histology
Introductory Physiology	Introductory Med Psyche	

M.D. Curriculum

The curriculum is conducted over a four-year program. For those with a Bachelor's degree or who have completed the premedical requirements, it can be completed in three years and four months. A five-year program is also available designed for high school graduates who have not yet completed prerequisite coursework. AUSM designs the curriculum to mirror the quality found in United States medical schools.

Basic Sciences

The basic sciences are conducted over the first two years on the Aruba campus and focus on developing the basic knowledge of health and disease. The Basic Sciences are followed immediately by the Introduction to Clinical Medicine program prior to entering the third year Clinical Clerkship rotations.

Basic Science Curriculum

Semester I	Semester II	Semester III	Semester IV	Semester V
Gross Anatomy	Biochemistry	Microbiology & Immunology	Pathology II	Introduction to Clinical Medicine
Histology	Physiology	Psychology	Epidemiology & Preventive Medicine	Board Review
Medical Embryology	Generics	Pathology I	Physical Diagnosis	
Medical Ethics	Neurosciences	Pharmacology		

Clinical Sciences

The Clinical Science clerkships are conducted primarily in the United States but can occur as well in India, the Caribbean, or Canada.

Clinical Science Curriculum

Required – 48 weeks		Electives - 24-30 weeks	
Internal Medicine	12 weeks	Orthopedics	Pathology
Surgery	12 weeks	Pediatrics	Ophthalmology
Pediatrics	6 weeks	ENT	OB/GYN
OB/GYN	6 weeks	Intensive Care	Urology
Psychiatry	6 weeks	Surgery	Endocrinology
Family Medicine	6 weeks	Psychiatry	many others

Grading

Students are promoted from one semester to the next after passing all courses for that semester and achieve graduation after satisfactorily meeting all performance standards. The exam schedule is rigorous and designed to help students remain focused. The Dean promotes a student into the clinical clerkship program only after completing all of the Basic Science program requirements. Successful completion of the Basic and Clinical Sciences as well as passing either USMLE® Step 1 or Step 2 (or the foreign equivalents) are required to be eligible for graduation.

ENTRANCE REQUIREMENTS:

Pre-Medical Program (5-year MD Program)

Requires the completion of a High School Diploma. Applicants must by United States or Canadian citizens.

M.D. Program

The minimum requirement for admission is 90 semester hours of college level courses. A baccalaureate degree is preferred and preference will be given to applicants who will have completed this prior to matriculation. College work must include the following (the successful completion of labs are expected with science courses nearly universally even when not specifically listed):

- General Biology or Zoology – one academic year
- General Inorganic Chemistry – one academic year
- Advance Chemistry – one academic year
- Physics – one academic year
- English – one academic year
- College Mathematics – one academic year

A broad background in the humanities and social sciences is recommended. The MCAT® is not currently required but is recommended. For applicants who have taken the MCAT®, submission of scores is expected.

SELECTION FACTORS:

Aureus University seeks students who have the strong desire for success and demonstrate the ability to be able to practice compassionate and humanitarian medicine. The greatest weight is placed on the scholastic record, but many other factors are taken into account as well. The interview is extremely important as is the educational level of the student and level of commitment. Students are expected to present a strong case for themselves by describing their scholastic achievements, community contributions, volunteer work, and must have three strong letters of recommendations. Applicants will be notified within two to three weeks of their acceptance status. There is no application deadline as the school operates under rolling admissions with classes starting in January, May, and September. The MCAT® is not required, but submission of MCAT® scores is expected if the test has been taken.

TUITION AND FINANCIAL AID:

Application Fee: $49 USD (non-refundable)

Admission/Enrollment Fee: $795 USD (non-refundable)

Payment required to secure acceptance: $795 USD

Tuition for 5-year MD Degree Program (3 semesters): $5,295 USD per semester

Tuition for Basic Sciences: $6,495 to $6,750 USD per semester

Tuition for Clinical Sciences: $7,995 USD per semester

Malpractice Insurance: $800-1200 USD per year

Lab fee: $250 one-time fee

Graduation Fee: $700

Other fees such as student and administrative may apply.

Five merit based scholarships are available for outstanding and deserving students and range from $2,500 to $5,000 USD each. Private loans are available. Private tuition loans are available to a select number of competitive students. United States Federal student loans are not available at this time.

ooooo

Xavier University School of Medicine

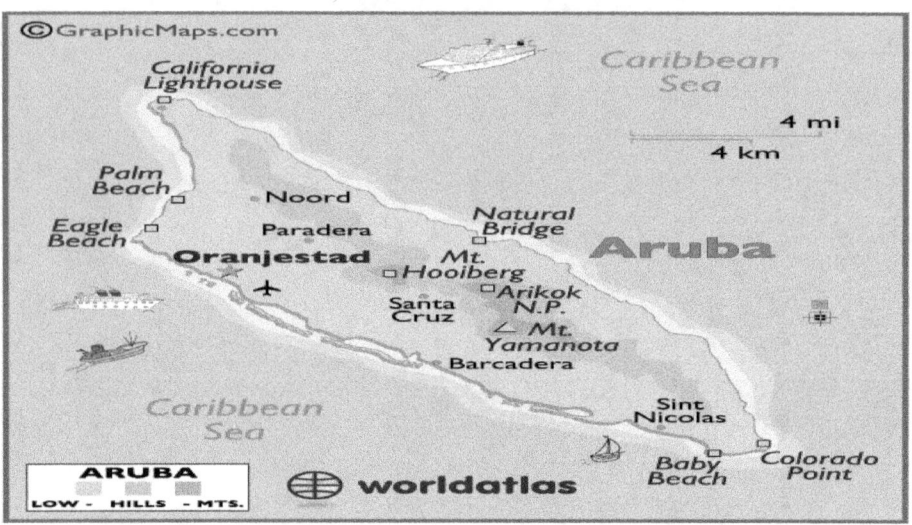

AMRCB® QUICK REFERENCE
Xavier University School of Medicine

Year Founded	2005	Currency	AWG
On-Campus Housing	No	Airport Code	AUA
Pre-Medical Program	Yes	Time Zone	EST (GMT/UTC-5)
MCAT® Required	No	Electricity	110 V
Official Language	Dutch	Driving Side	Right

Xavier University School of Medicine

Aruba

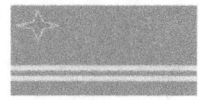

Ravishankar Bhooplapur - President
Edwin Casey - Chairman / Trustee
Burton L. Herx, M.D., F.A.C.S., F.A.C.G. - Dean of Clinical Sciences

CONTACT INFORMATION:

U.S. Admission Office
Xavier Admissions Aruba, LLC
1000 Woodbury Road, Suite 109
Woodbury, NY 11797 U.S.A.

Campus Address
Xavier University School of Medicine
Santa Helenastraat #23
Oranjestad, Aruba

General Information
Telephone: 526-333-2224
Fax: 516-921-1070
Website: http://www.xusom.com
E-Mail: info@xusom.com

GENERAL INFORMATION:

Xavier University School of Medicine (XUSOM) was founded in 2005. The curriculum is designed to be highly integrated, unique, and flexible for the purpose of developing knowledgeable, skillful, and compassionate physicians. XUSOM strives to keep the student faculty ratio at 25:1 allowing for an individuated learning environment.

The physical campus is newly renovated and modern with 125,000 square feet (11.600 m²) of state-of-the-art equipment. XUSOM distinguishes itself from other Caribbean medical schools in that the overall educational curriculum is accelerated and spans just over three years and is completed in 38 months. This is done without compromising clinical exposure or the total number of credited hours. This allows for the shortest duration of training of the medical schools located throughout the Caribbean. Students still have adequate time to pursue research, additional advanced degrees, or to participate in specialized tracks. The school operates under a rolling admissions system with three classes starting each year in January, May, and September.

XUSOM offers a traditional four-year MD program and a five and half year program for high school graduates. A three year Bachelor's in Nursing (BSN) degree is also offered and XUSOM participates in several international educational programs. Combined degrees are also available in cooperation with Walden University including a Master in Business Administration (MBA), Master of Healthcare Administration (MHA), and a Master in Public Health (MPH). Transfer students are considered. Campus housing is not currently available.

XUSOM is listed by the International Medical Education Directory (IMED), the World Health Organization (WHO), and is listed with the Medical Council of Canada (MCC). At the time of this publication, AUSOM has been provisionally accredited by the Caribbean Accreditation Authority for Education in Medicine and the Health Professions (CAAM-HP) but is not currently certified by the American Medical Residency Certification Board (AMRCB®). Students are eligible for ECFMG® certification. XUSOM is independently charted by the Government of Aruba of the Dutch Antilles.

CURRICULUM:

PRE-MEDICAL PROGRAM

The Premedical Program spans four semesters and focuses on the needed sciences to become prepared for the medical curriculum. Upon successful completion, students will automatically gain advancement into the Basic Sciences.

Pre-Medical Program

Semester I	Semester II	Semester III	Semester IV
General Biology	Biology and Genetics	Intro to Histology and Cell Biology	Intro to Biochemistry
General Chemistry	Behavioral Science	Medical Terminology	Intro to Microbiology
Calculus	Physics	Intro to Anatomy	Intro to Physiology
Medical Communication	General Chemistry	Organic Chemistry	Intro to Neuroanatomy

M.D. PROGRAM

The curriculum is conducted over a total time frame of 38 months. The Basic Sciences are conducted over five semesters which are the same for the traditional four-year program and the five and a half year program.

Basic Sciences

The Basic Sciences are conducted over five semesters which span 20 months on the medical campus in Aruba. This is followed by a sixth semester which serves as a transition into the Clinical Sciences.

Basic Science Curriculum

Semester I	Semester II	Semester III	Semester IV	Semester V
Fundamental Concepts	Nervous System	Gastro-intestinal System	Cardiovascular System	Renal and Metabolic System
Musculoskeletal System	Nutrition and Metabolism	Respiratory System	Hematopoietic System	Endocrine System
Patient, Doctor, and Society I	Patient, Doctor, and Society II	Patient, Doctor, and Society III	Patient, Doctor, and Society IV	Reproductive System
Healthcare Quality Improvement I	Healthcare Quality Improvement II	Healthcare Quality Improvement III	Healthcare Quality Improvement IV	Patient, Doctor, and Society V
				Healthcare Quality Improvement V

Clinical Sciences

The Clinical clerkships are conducted over six semesters which span 72 weeks primarily in the United States as well as Puerto Rico.

Clinical Science Curriculum

Required – 48 weeks		Electives – 24 weeks	
Internal Medicine	12 weeks	Emergency Medicine	Dermatology
Surgery	12 weeks	Medical Oncology	Pathology
Pediatrics	6 weeks	Radiology	Anesthesiology
OB/GYN	6 weeks	Cardiology	Immunology
Psychiatry	6 weeks	Gastroenterology	NICU
Family Medicine	6 weeks	Surgical	many others

Grading

Students are promoted from one semester to the next after passing all courses for that semester and achieve graduation after satisfactorily meeting all performance standards. A student is promoted into the clinical clerkship program only after completing all of the Basic Science program requirements.

ENTRANCE REQUIREMENTS:

Pre-Medical Program

Students must have a High School Diploma and a cumulative GPA of 3.0. The SAT or ACT must have been taken. SAT scores should be 1200 (old system) or 1800 (new system) and ACT scores should be 26 or higher. For students who are not native English speakers, they should have TOEFL® scores that are 231 or higher or an IELTS™ score that is 6.0 or greater.

MD Program

The minimum requirement for admission is 90 credits (semester) hours of college level courses with a cumulative Grade Point Average of 3.0. A baccalaureate degree is not required. College work must include the following:

- General Biology with Lab – one academic year
- Inorganic of General Chemistry with Lab – one academic year
- Organic Chemistry with Lab – one academic year
- Physics with Lab – one academic year
- English – 6 credit hours
- Pre-Calculus or Calculus – one academic year

The MCAT® is not required.

SELECTION FACTORS:

The school has an open admissions system and advanced standing is considered for transfer applicants. Exposure to clinical medicine whether in a volunteer setting or other clinical setting is important prior to applying to medical school, however, volunteer experience is not required for admission. The average GPA of accepted students is 3.2. Interviews are conducted by phone or via Skype video conference. There is no application deadline as the school operates under a rolling admissions system with classes starting in January, May, and September each year. The MCAT® is not required for admission, but students who have taken the MCAT® are encouraged to submit scores. Once accepted, students are assigned a faculty advisor to aid with guidance on academic and personal issues, as well as overall adjustment to life in Aruba.

TUITION AND FINANCIAL AID:

Application Fee: $75 USD (non-refundable)

New Students Registration Fee: $700 USD

Payment required to secure acceptance: $1000 USD (non-refundable)

Tuition for Pre-Medical Program (semesters 1-4): $5,000 USD per semester

Tuition for Basic Sciences: $8,400 USD per semester

Tuition for Sixth Semester: $10,800 USD

Tuition for Clinical Sciences: $10,800 USD per semester

Student Administrative Fee: $528 USD per semester

Graduation Fee: $600 USD

Malpractice Insurance: $1,200 USD per clinical year

Other fees such as laboratory, exam, and student may apply.

Merit based scholarships, payment plans, and private loans are available. Students who have taken the MCAT® are encouraged to submit scores as several specific scholarships are available and based directly on MCAT® scores and GPA's. Scholarships are also available for transfer students and based on USMLE® scores. United States Federal student loans are not available at this time.

○○○○○

AURBA INFORMATION

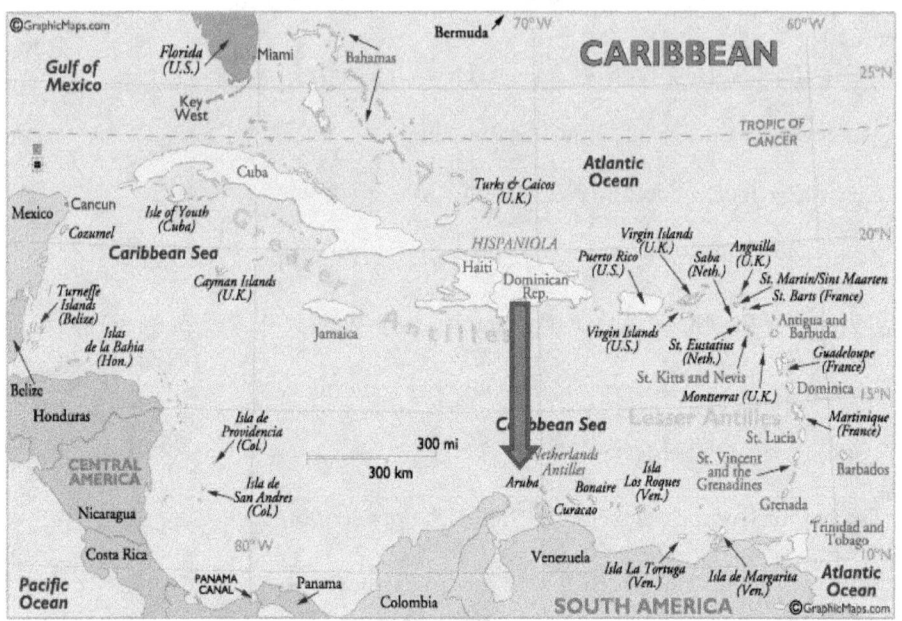

Aruba is located in the West Indies 15 miles (24 km) off the coast of Venezuela and has been under Spanish and Dutch possession throughout history. The island has an area of 75 square miles (194 km²) and is 19 miles (30 km) long and 5 miles (8 km) wide. The capital, Oranjestad, has a population of 20,000 and the entire population of Aruba is 66,687 persons. Xavier University and Aureus are both located in Oranjestad.

Aruba had been a member of the Netherlands-Antilles until 1986 when it became an autonomous and self-governing island. The official head of government is the Dutch monarch and defense of the island is the official responsibility of the Netherlands. Dutch is the official language, but every Aruban child studies

English and Spanish from the age of ten so most residents speak these languages as well. A local dialect, Papiamento, is also spoken and is a language that has evolved over the centuries from a mixture of Spanish, Dutch, and Portuguese. Roman Catholicism and Anglican religions are predominant on the island.

The average daytime temperature is 82°F (27°C) and the island is kept cool by the trade winds. The difference between median day and night temperatures, and between summer and winter temperatures, is just 3.6°F (2°C). The humidity is low and the average annual rainfall is 24 inches (609 mm). The rainfall occurs mainly in short showers during October, November, and December. Aruba lies outside of the hurricane belt.

Historically, petroleum had been the primary industry for the island. Aruba now depends primarily on tourism and the export of tobacco and consumer goods. The currency is the Aruban guilder (AWG) with an exchange rate of 1.00 USD to 1.79 AWG. The time zone is the same as the Eastern Standard Time in the United States and is 5 hours behind Greenwich Mean Time. Electricity is 110 volts which is the same as in the United States.

Aruba is accessed through the Queen Beatrix International Airport (AUA). Flights are available from the United States on Air ALM, American Airlines, Martinair, Continental, Delta, TWA, Vacation Express, and charter flights. Flights from Canada are available on U.S. Airways, Delta, Canada 3000, Air Transit, Air Canada, American Airlines, and Continental. Flights are also available from the United Kingdom, Holland, South America, and throughout the Caribbean. Driving is on the right hand side of the road just as in North America.

ooooo

Central and South American Medical Schools - Caribbean Region

Saint James School of Medicine Bonaire

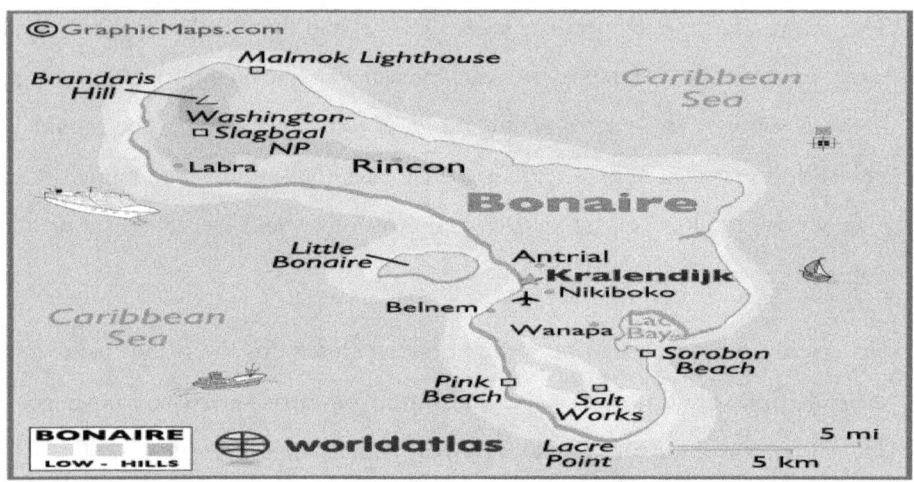

AMRCB® QUICK REFERENCE
Saint James School of Medicine

Year Founded	1999	Currency	USD
On-Campus Housing	No	Airport Code	BON
Pre-Medical Program	No	Time Zone	AST (GMT/UTC-4)
MCAT® Required	No	Electricity	110 V
Official Language	Dutch	Driving Side	Right

Saint James School of Medicine – Bonaire

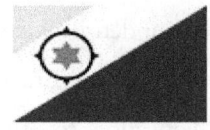

Samam Bentota - Faculty
Dr. Gawande - Faculty

CONTACT INFORMATION:

U.S. Admissions Office
Saint James School of Medicine
c/o Human Resource Development Services (HDRS) Inc.
1480 Renaissance Drive, Suite 300
Parke Ridge, Illinois U.S.A.   60068

Campus Address
Saint James School of Medicine
Plaza Juliana 4
Kralendijk, Bonaire

General Information
Telephone: 800-542-1553
Fax: 847-298-2539
Website: http://bonaire.sjsm.org/
E-Mail: info@mail.sjsm.org

GENERAL INFORMATION:

Saint James School of Medicine (SJSM) was initially founded in 1999 with the first medical school class starting in 2001 and has been in continuous operation since that time. St. James has campuses on Bonaire, Anguilla, and on Saint Vincent. The first campus was opened on Bonaire in 1999 and began instruction in 2000. The second campus was opened in Anguilla in 2010, with the Saint Vincent campus opening in 2014. Over 2,500 students have matriculated into the institution. Saint James was founded by a consortium of medical educators and physician from the United States and Europe with the goal of offering high quality, affordable medical education to students from the United States and Canada. The mission is to assist motivated students in becoming successful physicians with a commitment to problem solving, and the well-being of their patients and society.

The Bonaire campus was slated for closure in 2013 with all students being transferred to the Anguilla campus. New requirements by the Government of the Netherlands resulted in the potential de-listing of the school from the International Medical Directory. Even if the IMED were to de-list the school, the World Health Directory and other recognitions would not be affected. At this time of this publication, it is reported that the Bonaire campus will be able to remain open.

The curriculum is modeled after the United States medical school educational system and spans ten semesters. The curriculum is designed around problem-based learning and focused on preparing students for the USMLE® examinations. Students will learn and practice how to understand research methods, how to develop a hypothesis, and to think critically during the Basic Sciences. No on-campus student is currently available, although St. James does have a housing coordinator that assists students in securing housing. Housing costs approximate $800 USD per month depending on occupancy and amenities. A Pre-Medical program was available on the Bonaire campus in the past but is no longer available.

Saint James can only accept applications from United States citizens or permanent residents, or from Canadian citizens. Saint James does accept transfer students on an individual basis into the Basic Science and Clinical Science phases. In general, students must be transferring from an accredited medical school. No application deadline exists as the school operates under a rolling admissions system. Currently, there are three starting classes each year in January, May, and September.

Saint James is recognized by the ECFMG® and is currently listed in the International Medical Directory by FAIMER®. SJSM is listed by the World Health Organization (WHO), accredited by the Caribbean Authority for Education in Medicine and other Health Professions (CAAM-HP), and accredited by the Medical Council of Canada. Saint James is not certified by the AMRCB® at the time of publication. In addition, Saint James is recognized by the Israeli Ministry of Health and accredited by the governments of Bonaire, Anguilla, and Saint Vincent.

CURRICULUM:

The curriculum is conducted over a four-year program consisting of 10 semesters that are each four months long. The four-year program can be completed in as little as three years and six months although most students complete the program over four years. The Basic Sciences are conducted over four semesters on the clinical campus on Bonaire and the Clinical Science rotations take place over six semesters at affiliated facilities in the United States. The entire curriculum is based on problem-solving techniques which are designed to assist students in preparing for the USMLE®.

In addition to the Basic and Clinical Science rotations, students must demonstrate proficiency in medical research in order to graduate. Research begins during the Basic Science rotations and continues through the Clinical Science rotations. Students are able to select a research project from their own areas of interest in basic, clinical, or applied science. Saint James states that a strong research project will aid students in presenting and understanding scientific information and strengthen a student's residency application.

Basic Sciences

The Basic Sciences take place over 16 months on the Bonaire campus. All courses are designed in the USMLE® format and integrated with hands on clinical training when possible.

Basic Science Curriculum

Semester I	Semester II	Semester III	Semester IV
Histology	Physiology	Pathology I	Pathology II
Gross Anatomy and Embryology	Biochemistry	Microbiology	Epidemiology and Biostatistics
Embryology	Neurosciences	Pharmacology	Physical Diagnosis and Clinical Medicine
Medical and Legal Ethics	Genetics	Medical Psychology	Research in Health and Medicine II
Clinical Correlation of Basic Science I	Research in Health and Medicine I	Research in Health and Medicine II	Clinical Correlation of Basic Science IV
	Clinical Correlation of Basic Science II	Clinical Correlation of Basic Science III	

Clinical Sciences

The Clinical clerkships are conducted primarily in the United States and take place over six semesters consisting of 96 weeks. The clinical clerkships are currently held in various locations including Illinois, West Virginia, and Arizona. All rotations are arranged by Saint James.

Training in clinical medicine begins with a structured course entitled "Advanced Introduction to Clinical Medicine." This course is conducted in Chicago and takes place over eight weeks and consists of an intensive USMLE® Step 1 review followed by eight weeks of an introduction to clinical medicine in various clinical departments. This introductory course allows medical students to have acquired basic clinical skills prior to officially starting clinical rotations.

Clinical Science Curriculum

Required - 48 Weeks		Electives - 48 Weeks	
Internal Medicine	12 weeks	Nephrology	Urology
Surgery	12 weeks	Infectious Disease	Surgical
Pediatrics	6 weeks	Hematology	Rheumatology
OB/GYN	6 weeks	Gastroenterology	Radiology
Psychiatry	6 weeks	Dermatology	Emergency Medicine
Family Medicine	6 weeks	Orthopedics	many others

Grading

Students are promoted from one semester to the next after passing all courses for that semester and achieve graduation after satisfactorily meeting all performance standards. The Dean promotes a student into the clinical clerkship program only after completing all of the Basic Science program requirements and passing USMLE® Step 1. Students must demonstrate proficiency in medical research in order to be eligible for graduation.

ENTRANCE REQUIREMENTS:

The minimum requirement for admission is 90 semester hours (three years) of college level courses. A baccalaureate degree is preferred and preference will be given to applicants who will have completed this prior to matriculation. Completion of standard pre-medical science coursework is expected. The MCAT® is not required for admission.

SELECTION FACTORS:

The school has an open admissions system and advanced standing is considered for transfer applicants. Saint James can only accept applications from United States citizens or permanent residents, or from Canadian citizens. Prospective students are evaluated on a number of factors including the undergraduate GPA, letters of recommendation, prior course work, volunteer/work experience, the personal essay, the interview, and individual student motivations. Students who have a lower GPA are expected to have strong letters of recommendation. Applicants will be notified of a decision within three weeks of their acceptance status. No application deadline is in place as the school operates under a rolling admissions system with classes starting in January, May, and September. Students can reserve a place in any of the starting semesters.

TUITION AND FINANCIAL AID:

Application Fee: $75 USD

Enrollment Fee: $2,000 USD (non-refundable). This does include $1000 USD to secure acceptance which is applied to tuition.

Tuition for Basic Sciences: $5,500 USD per semester

Tuition for Advanced Introduction to Clinical Medicine: $8,200 USD

Tuition for Clinical Sciences: $ 8,200 USD per semester

Annual liability insurance during the clinical years: $800 USD per year

Other fees such as laboratory, student, administrative, and graduation may apply.

Merit based scholarships, student credit lines, and private loans are available. Delta student loans are utilized by many students. United States Federal student loans are not currently available. Payment plans are available for students who meet specific requirements.

ooooo

BONAIRE INFORMATION

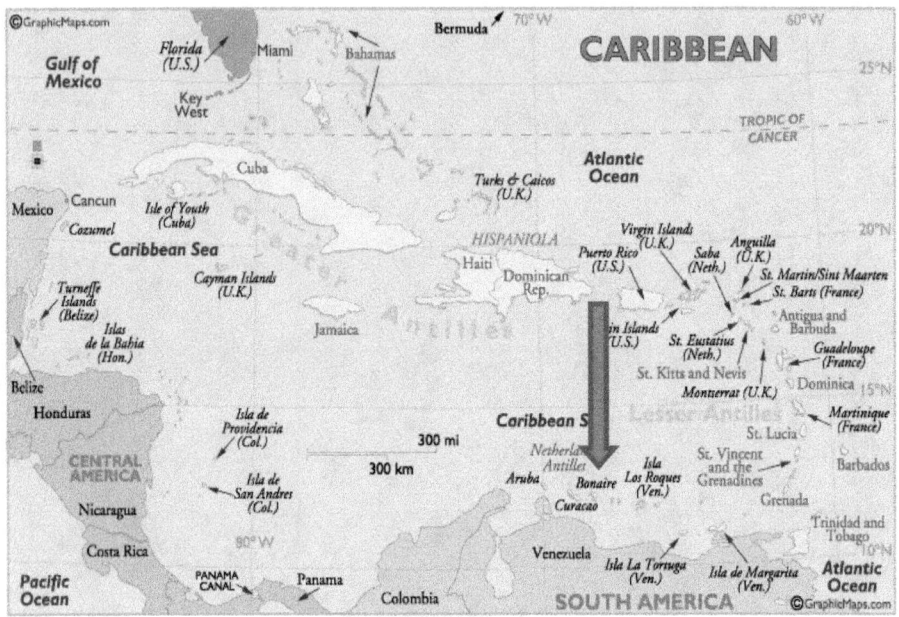

Bonaire is in the southern Caribbean and is part of the Netherlands Antilles located off the coast of Venezuela. Bonaire is located 50 miles (80 km) north of Venezuela, and 30 miles (48 km) east of Curacao. The island has an area of 112 square miles (288 km²) with the highest point of 784 feet (240 m) on Mount Brandaris. The island has a population of 17,500 and the capital and largest city is Kralendijk. The St. James campus is located in Kralendijk. The majority of the population is indigenous to the Netherland Antilles.

Bonaire, along with the uninhabited islet of Klein Bonaire, forms a special municipality of the Netherlands. Bonaire was part of the Netherlands Antilles until the country's dissolution in 2010. The county had been controlled by the

Dutch, Spanish, and English historically and was controlled by Germany during World War II. Dutch is the official language although only spoken by only 9% of the population. Papiamento (a creole dialect) is officially recognized also and spoken by 75% of the population. Nearly all residents speak English or Spanish in public. Bonaire is known for scuba diving, snorkeling, and windsurfing with tourism serving at the primary industry of the island.

The island lies outside of the hurricane belt and has not been struck by a hurricane for the last 70 years. The average daily temperature is 80°F (27°C) with constant easterly trade winds keeping the island cool. The average humidity is 75% with an average rainfall of 22 inches (560 mm) a year.

The official currency is now the U.S. dollar having recently switched from the NAFL (Guilder). The time zone is Atlantic Standard Time which is four hours behind GMT and one hour ahead of Eastern Standard Time. The primary religion is Christianity with the only active churches on the island being of the Christian denomination. Electricity is standard at 110 volts/60 cycles just as in North America.

Air travel is through the Flamingo International Airport (BON) on Bonaire. Bonaire is served by domestic and international airlines including American Airlines, Air Jamaica, Antilles Air, United Airlines, Delta Air Lines, KLM, and Insel Airlines. Connections are available out of Aruba, Curacao, and Venezuela. The majorities of transfers fly from Curacao and take the ten minute flight to Bonaire via Insel Air. Driving is on the right hand side of the road just as in North America and the island does not have any traffic lights.

ooooo

Avalon University School of Medicine

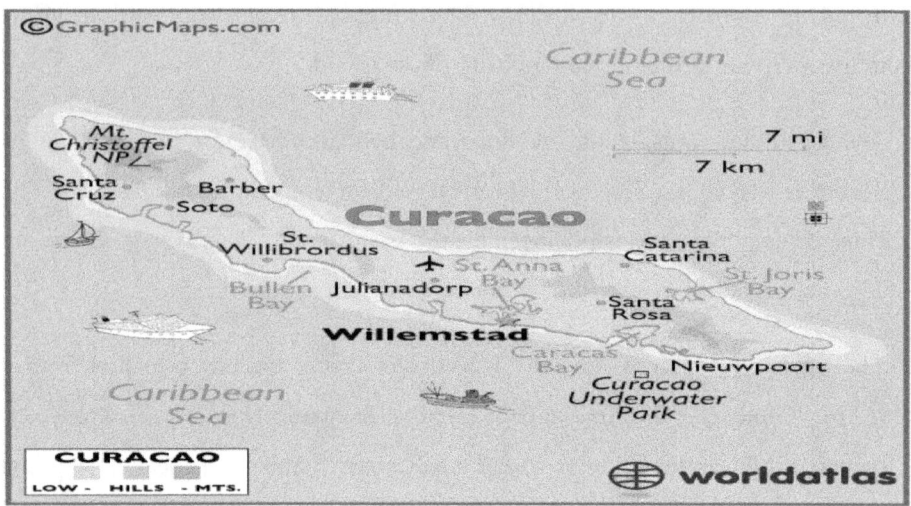

AMRCB® QUICK REFERENCE
Avalon University School of Medicine

Year Founded	2003	Currency	ANG
On-Campus Housing	Yes (limited)	Airport Code	CUR
Pre-Medical Program	Yes	Time Zone	AST (GMT/UTC-4)
MCAT® Required	No	Electricity	120/127 V
Official Language	Dutch, English, and Papiamentu	Driving Side	Right

Avalon University School of Medicine

Curacao

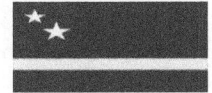

Shokat Fattey, M.D. - Chancellor
Samir Fatteh, M.D. - President
John Nekic, M.D. - Executive Dean

CONTACT INFORMATION:

U.S. Admission Office
Avalon University School of Medicine
P.O Box 480
Girard, OH 44420 U.S.A.

Campus Address
Avalon University School of Medicine
Scharlooweg 25
Willemstad, Curacao
Netherlands Antilles

Indian Admissions Office
#204, 2nd Floor - Bhanu Towers
Opposite ESI Hospital
Errgadda Hyderabad
Andhra Pradesh 500018
Phone: +91 40-23714565, 9177734565

General Information
Telephone: 1-855-282-5668 or
             330- 759-8008
Fax: 330-759-8041
Website: http://www.avalonu.org
E-Mail: admissions@avalonu.org

GENERAL INFORMATION:

Avalon University School of Medicine (AUSOM) was founded in 2003. The mission is to educate students in the art and science of medicine and to promote growth and learning, dedication, discipline, and direction. AUSOM encourages participation in social and community activities and maintains a small class size of 25 students per class.

The school focuses on quality medical education with a curriculum that focuses on preparing students for the USMLE® examinations. Hands-on learning is coupled with theoretical knowledge and live patient presentations to develop effective clinicians. The medical school follows the North American educational model and guarantees clinical rotations in the United States for students who desire this. A Master of Business Administration (M.B.A.) and Master of Healthcare Administration (M.H.A.) degrees are available as dual degrees for those interested in cooperation with Davenport University, Walden University, and Drexel University. Research opportunities are available for interested students as well.

AUSUM offers pre-medical programs in Curacao, Chicago, and Ontario which guarantee acceptance into the medical school for students who have completed the program with certain academic requirements. The campus has recently secured land to build a new campus on the island of Curacao. AUSOM offers limited on-campus student housing at this time for 15 students and assists other students in finding housing. A student dress code is in place. Transfer students are considered. There is no application deadline as the school operates under a rolling admissions system with classes starting in January, May, and September each year.

AUSUM is listed by the International Medical Education Directory (IMED), the World Health Organization (WHO), and the Medical Council of Canada (MCC). At the time of this publication, St. Matthew's is not currently certified by the American Medical Residency Certification Board (AMRCB®). Students are eligible for ECFMG® certification. AUSUM is chartered by the Ministry of Education in Curacao

CURRICULUM:

Pre-Medical Program

The Pre-Medical program develops the necessary foundation for students to begin the accelerated, advanced studies needed in the medical sciences. Students who successfully complete the coursework will automatically gain advancement into the four-year M.D. program. Avalon has three Pre-Medical programs offered in the following locations: Northwest Suburban College in Rolling Meadows, Illinois (12 miles outside of Chicago); Ontario, Canada; and on the Curacao campus.

The program at Northwest Suburban College involves 20 months of study and students are awarded an Associate of Science degree at completion which satisfactorily meets the prerequisites for the Avalon M.D. program.

The program in Mississauga, Ontario is affiliated with Biztech College. Students are able to complete all the pre-medical requirements over one year which then allows promotion into the Avalon M.D. program.

The Curacao program is offered on the Avalon campus allowing students to complete the prerequisites and then directly enter the M.D. program.

Pre-Medical Curacao Curriculum

Semester I	Semester II	Semester III	Semester IV
General Biology I	General Biology II	Intro to Histology and Cell Biology	Intro to Anatomy and Physiology
General Chemistry I	General Chemistry II	Organic Chemistry I	Organic Chemistry II
Pre-Calculus	Calculus	General Physics I	General Physics II
English I	English II	Psychology	Ethics
			Medical Terminology

M.D. Curriculum

Basic Sciences

The Basic Sciences take place over 16 months on the campus in Curacao. A fifth semester takes place in Beckley, West Virginia over 16 weeks and is designed to be a bridge between the Basic Medical Sciences and the Clinical Sciences. The fifth semester includes the following courses: Introduction to Clinical Medicine, Getting into Residency, and a Kaplan Review. The fifth semester also covers multiple needed certifications required to start clinical medicine.

Basic Science Curriculum

Semester I	Semester II	Semester III	Semester IV
Medical Embryology	Neuroscience	Pathology I	Pathology II
Biostatistics and Epidemiology I	Biochemistry	Behavioral Sciences and Medical Ethics	Pharmacology
Gross Anatomy	Medical Physiology	Medical Microbiology & Immunology	Physical Diagnosis
Histology, Cell, and Molecular Biology	Genetics		Intro to Clinical Medicine and EBM

Clinical Sciences

The Clinical clerkships are conducted over 72 weeks primarily in the United States and begin after the fifth semester. Students are able to arrange their own clinical rotations if desired.

Clinical Science Curriculum

Required – 48 weeks		Electives – 24 weeks	
Internal Medicine	12 - weeks	Cardiology	Otolaryngology
Surgery	12 - weeks	Radiology	Gastroenterology
Pediatrics	6 - weeks	Pulmonology	Neurology
OB/GYN	6 - weeks	Hematology	Oncology
Psychiatry	6 - weeks	Dermatology	Orthopedics
Family Medicine	6 - weeks	Pediatric	many others

Grading

Students are promoted from one semester to the next after passing all courses for that semester and achieve graduation after satisfactorily meeting all performance standards. The Dean promotes a student into the clinical clerkship program only after completing all of the Basic Science program requirements.

ENTRANCE REQUIREMENTS:

Pre-Medical Program

Students must have graduated High School to be eligible for each program. Each individual program will have specific individual requirements.

M.D. Program

The minimum requirement for admission is 90 semester hours of college level courses or a baccalaureate degree or equivalent prior to matriculation. Exceptions will be considered on an individual basis. College work must include the following (the successful completion of labs are expected with science courses nearly universally even when not specifically listed):

- General Biology, Anatomy, or Zoology – one academic year
- General/Inorganic Chemistry – one academic year
- Biochemistry/Organic Chemistry – one academic year
- Physics – one academic year
- English – one academic year
- Calculus – one course

A broad background in the humanities, social sciences or physical sciences, and computer skills are recommended. The MCAT® is not required.

SELECTION FACTORS:

The school has an open admissions system and advanced standing is considered for transfer applicants. Interviews are conducted via phone and the personal interview is a large part of the selection process. AUSOM seeks students with maturity, a concern for others, integrity, and those that display leadership potential. The University is interested in why students want to become doctors, what experiences have lead them to this career, and the ability of students to handle the rigorous academic challenges of medical school. The applicant's academic record, essay, extracurricular activities, and letters of recommendation will all be considered. MCAT® scores are not required but can be submitted if taken.

There is no application deadline as the school operates under a rolling admissions system with classes starting in January, May, and September each year. Students can apply to any semester. It can take up to three months for immigration paperwork for the island of Curacao to be completed so this must be considered when selecting a starting date.

TUITION AND FINANCIAL AID:

Application Fee: $50 USD (non-refundable)

Admission Fee: $900 USD

Payment required to secure acceptance: $1,000 USD (non-refundable)

Tuition for Pre-Medical Program (semesters 1-4): $4,500 per semester

Tuition for Basic Sciences: $6,500 USD per semester

Fifth Semester: $7,700 USD

Tuition for Clinical Sciences: $7,700 USD per semester
(Some Clinical Rotation sites may require additional surcharges)

Graduation Fee: $500 USD

Laboratory Fee: $350 USD

Other fees such as student, administrative, and Government may apply.

Merit based scholarships and private loans are available. United States Federal student loans are not available at this time.

No immigration fee is in place for the island, although a refundable deposit of $571 - $3143 USD depending on the country of citizenship is required.

ooooo

Caribbean Medical University School of Medicine

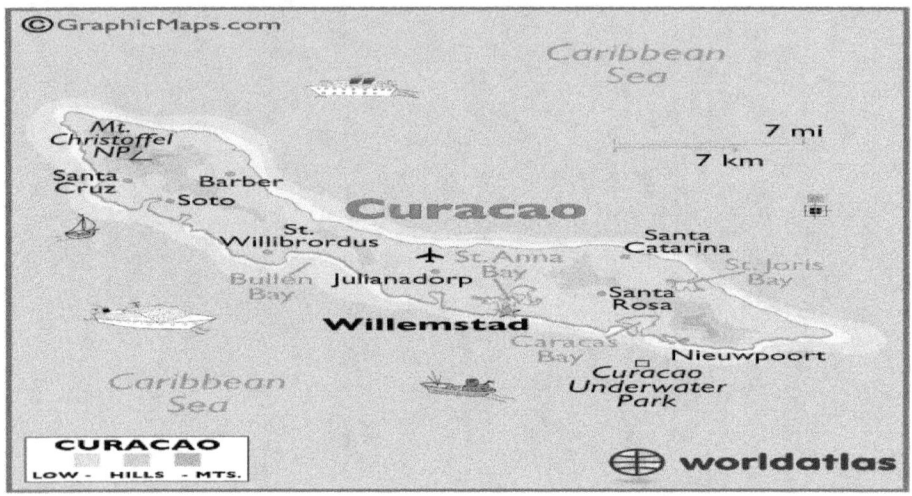

AMRCB® QUICK REFERENCE
Caribbean Medical University School of Medicine

Year Founded	2007	Currency	ANG
On-Campus Housing	Yes	Airport Code	CUR
Pre-Medical Program	Yes	Time Zone	AST (GMT/UTC-4)
MCAT® Required	No	Electricity	120/127 V
Official Language	Dutch, English, and Papiamentu	Driving Side	Right

Caribbean Medical University School of Medicine

Curacao

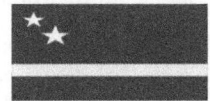

Ryan Jackson, M.D., M.S. - Dean of Academics
Sunny Handa, M.D. - Dean of Clinical Medicine (Teaching Physician)

CONTACT INFORMATION:

U.S. Admission Office
Caribbean Medical University
5600 North River Road - Suite 800
Chicago, Illinois 60018, USA
Tel: 1-888-877-4268
Fax: 1-302-397-2092
Email: info@cmumed.org
Web: www.cmumed.org

Main Campus
WTC Piscadera Bay
Willemstad, Curacao
Tel: 1-888-877-4268
Fax: 1-302-397-2092
Email: info@cmumed.org
Web: www.cmumed.org

Canadian Admissions Office
Caribbean Medical University
2425 Matheson Boulevard East – 8th Floor
Mississauga, Ontario – L4W 5K4, Canada
Tel: 1-877-517-8800
Fax: 1-480-772-4409
Email: canada@cmumed.org
Web: www.cmumed.org

Satellite Premedical Program Campuses
(Trillium-Academic-Program)
Mississauga, Ontario - Canada
Brampton, Ontario - Canada
Surrey, British Columbia - Canada
Calgary, Alberta - Canada

GENERAL INFORMATION:

The Caribbean Medical University (CMU) was founded in 2007 and seeks to be a transformational agent in healthcare while maintaining the highest possible standards. The average class size is small at 36 students with a teacher/student ratio at 16:1 optimizing the interaction and learning during classes. CMU bases the educational curriculum on the United States model and directly works to prepare students for the USMLE® examinations. The goal of the medical school is to prepare students to become practicing physicians and leaders in medicine by incorporating knowledge, comprehension, analysis, application, synthesis, and evaluation throughout the educational journey. Stated core values of the institution are integrity, teamwork, innovation, excellence, leadership, and professionalism. CMU works to identify and implement appropriate learning strategies for students to understand the social context of medicine.

CMU is housed in the World Trade Center (WTC) in Willemstad, which is one of the largest facilities on Curacao. The WTC is a 66,000 square foot (20,000 m^2) facility with a 400-seat auditorium, 19 classrooms, a computer lab, bank, restaurants, and a guest hotel. On-campus student housing is available in three different resident halls and additional housing is currently being built with costs ranging from $1600-$6000 USD per semester depending on amenities and occupancy. Transfer students are considered. There is no application deadline as the school operates under a rolling admissions system with classes starting in January, May, and September each year

Dual degrees are available for interested students including a Master in Public Health (M.P.H.) and a Master of Business Administration (M.B.A.) in cooperation with Walden University and Davenport University. In addition, CMU has numerous affiliations with other organizations across the international community. A Pre-Medical program is also available for motivated high school students that guarantees acceptance into the medical school after successful completion of prerequisite coursework. The average USMLE® pass-rate is currently 82%.

CMU is certified by the American Medical Residency Certification Board (AMRCB®) and is listed by the International Medical Education Directory (IMED), the World Health Organization (WHO), and recognized by the Medical Council of Canada (MCC). Students are eligible for ECFMG® certification. The Ministry of Education in Curacao charters CMU.

CURRICULUM:

Pre-Medical Sciences

The one-year Pre-Medical Program can be conducted at CMU's satellite campuses in Canada (Toronto – Ontario, Vancouver – British Columbia, Calgary – Alberta) or on the island for all three semesters. Students will get an approved Diploma of Premedical Sciences upon completion.

Pre-Medical Curriculum

Semester I	Semester II	Semester III
Calculus	Organic Chemistry I	Organic Chemistry II
General Chemistry	Cell Biology and Histology	English Composition
Evidence Based Research	Physics I	Physics II
Community Health and Wellness	Evidence Based Research	Medical Terminology
	Community Health and Wellness	Intro to Human Anatomy and Physiology
		Evidence Based Research
		Community Health and Wellness

M.D. Program

The curriculum is conducted via a trimester system over 10 semesters during the four-year program. Each semester is 16 weeks long. The Basic Sciences are conducted over the first four semesters, followed by a transitional fifth semester that prepares students for the clinical science rotations. CMU utilizes problem-based learning and includes case studies early in the curriculum. Patient contact begins early in the first year and includes clinical skills practice, patient simulations, physical diagnosis, and interviewing skills. The clinical experiences are conducted in three hospitals located on Curacao.

The 5-year Premedical/Doctor of Medicine Program (for high school graduates): The premedical sciences program is one-year in length and is conducted in a trimester system over 3 semesters. Each semester is 16 weeks long. High school graduates needing to acquire basic introductory knowledge prior to entering the M.D. program must complete a one-year premedical sciences program before advancing to the 4-year MD program. CMU's Premedical Program provides a basic foundation for courses including anatomy, physiology, histology, medical terminology, and others.

Basic Sciences

The first two academic years are conducted on Curacao during the first four semesters.

Basic Sciences Curriculum

Semester I	Semester II	Semester III	Semester IV	Semester V USMLE® Review
Gross Anatomy	Physiology	Pathology I	Pathology II	Cardiovascular, Pulmonology, and Hematology
Histology	Biochemistry	Microbiology / Immunology	Pharmacology	Neural and Musculoskeletal Sciences
Embryology	Biostatistics / Epidemiology	Neuroscience	Physical Diagnosis	Renal and Gastroenterology
	Genetics	Behavioral Sciences	Medical and Legal Ethics	Endocrinology and Reproductive Biology
				Hematology, Immunology, and Microbiology

Clinical Sciences

The Clinical Science clerkships are conducted over six semesters that span 72 weeks. Clinical rotations occur primarily in the United States and can occur in Canada as well as the United Kingdom. In the fifth semester during the clinical science transition, a USMLE® review program is taught in Champaign, Illinois or

Chicago, Illinois over a 15-week period. Clinical rotations begin after the successful completion of USMLE® Step 1.

Clinical Sciences Curriculum

Required – 48 weeks		Electives – 24 weeks	
Internal Medicine	12 - weeks	Anesthesiology	Cardiology
Surgery	12 - weeks	Critical Care	Cytology
Pediatrics	6 - weeks	Dermatology	Emergency Medicine
OB/GYN	6 - weeks	Geriatrics	Nephrology
Psychiatry	6 - weeks	Oncology	Pathology
Family Medicine	6 - weeks	Plastic Surgery	many others

Grading

Pre-medical and Basic Sciences courses in the first two and/or three years are evaluated on a percentage basis. Therefore, the student must not only pass the final exam but they must also complete all internal tests and assignments throughout the course. A minimum total grade of 60% is to be achieved to receive a pass and a credit for that course. In the third and fourth year, clinical clerkships are evaluated using **Caribbean Medical University's** clinical evaluation form. Students receive a grade out of 65 and are marked by the preceptor in 13 categories scoring a minimum of 0 to a maximum of 5 in each category. Students are also required to complete clinical case write-ups and daily logbooks for each clinical encounter during the clerkship. The preceptor must sign off and approve the case write-ups and logbooks. The students also conduct a 50-question multiple choice end of rotation clinical test, which contributes to a portion of the students clinical grade in the clerkship.

ENTRANCE REQUIREMENTS:

Pre-Medical Program

For high school graduates to gain admission into the Pre-Medical Program they must complete the following high school level courses:

- Grade 12 Biology
- Grade 12 Chemistry
- Grade 12 English
- Grade 12 Mathematics (Calculus, Computer Science, or Statistics)

Students must have a GPA of 2.8 or higher or a TOEFL® score of 60 or higher or IELTS™ score of 6.0 or higher. Students with an overall GPA of less than 2.8 must have strong letters of reference.

M.D. Program

The minimum requirement for admission into the MD program is 90 semester hours of postsecondary level courses. A baccalaureate degree or the equivalent is obtained by the majority of matriculated students but not required. College work must include the following (the successful completion of labs are expected with science courses nearly universally even when not specifically listed):

- General Biology or Zoology- one academic year

- General Chemistry – one academic year
- Organic Chemistry – one academic year
- General Physics – one academic year
- English – one semester
- Mathematics (Calculus, Computer Science, or Statistics) – one semester

The MCAT® is not required but applicants are highly encouraged to submit scores if the test is taken. If applicable, a TOEFL® score of 60, or an IELTS™ score of 6.0 is required.

SELECTION FACTORS:

The school has an open admissions system and advanced standing is considered for transfer applicants. A minimum GPA of 2.8 is expected as are strong letters of recommendation. Applicants will be assessed on their overall motivation to practice medicine. Personal interviews are requested at the discretion of the Admissions Committee. All applicants will be evaluated on an individual basis.

CMU seeks to identify the following strengths in potential applicants: observation skills; communication skills; motor skills; intellectual-conceptual ability; integrative and quantitative abilities; and behavioral and social attributes. Applicants will be notified within two weeks following their interview of their acceptance status. There is no application deadline as the school operates under a rolling admissions system with classes starting in January, May, and September each year. It can take up to three months for immigration paperwork for the island of Curacao to be completed so this must be considered when selecting a starting date.

TUITION AND FINANCIAL AID:

Application Fee: $75 USD (non-refundable)

Payment required securing acceptance: $1,000 USD

Tuition for Pre-Medical Sciences (4 semesters): $3,900 USD per semester

Tuition for Basic Sciences (4 semesters): $5,900 USD per semester

Tuition for Fifth Semester: $5,900 USD

Tuition Clinical Sciences (4 semesters): $7,900 USD per semester

Student Government Fee: $40 USD per semester

Graduation fee: $250 USD

Other fees such as laboratory, student, and administrative may apply.

Several merit-based scholarships are available with some scholarships covering up to 50% of tuition. Several private loans and tuition payment plans are also available. United States Federal student loans are not available at this time.

No immigration fee is in place for the island, although a refundable deposit of $571-$3143 USD depending on the country of citizenship is required.

○○○○○

St. Martinus University Faculty of Medicine

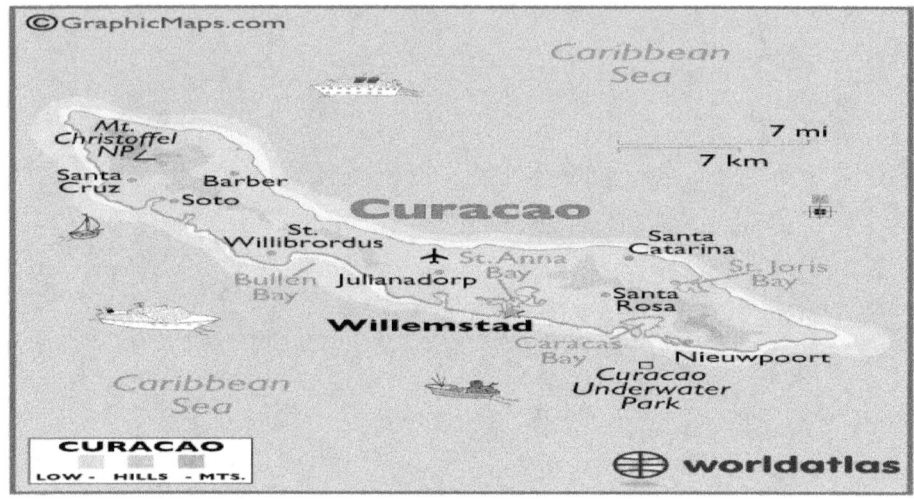

AMRCB® QUICK REFERENCE
St. Martinus University Faculty of Medicine

Year Founded	2000	Currency	ANG
On-Campus Housing	Yes	Airport Code	CUR
Pre-Medical Program	Yes	Time Zone	AST (GMT/UTC-4)
MCAT® Required	No	Electricity	120/127 V
Official Language	Dutch, English, and Papiamentu	Driving Side	Right

St. Martinus University Faculty of Medicine

Curacao

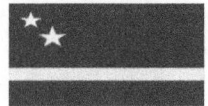

Dr. Sanjay Sharma - President
Kalcharan Misra, M.D., F.R.C.S., Ph.D. - Dean of Academics
James R. Brown, M.D. - Dean of Clinical Sciences

CONTACT INFORMATION:

U.S. Admission Office
St. Martinus University
8716 N. Mopac Expressway
Suite 20, Austin, TX 78759 U.S.A.

Campus Address
St. Martinus University
Kaya Fraternan di Skerpene #1
Scherpenheuvel, Willemstad, Curacao

Canada Admission Office
St. Martinus University
Unit #210
7990 Kennedy Rd. South
Brampton, Ontario, Canada L6W OB3
Telephone: (905) 867-3100

Asia Admission Office
St. Martinus Administrative Services
A-68, Sector-57
Noida, U.P. – 201301, India
Telephone: 0120-4782311;
084471-20255

General Information:
Telephone: 1-877-681-4SMU or 1-718-841-7682
Fax: 718-732-2503
Website: http://www.martinus.edu
E-Mail: admissions@martinus.edu

GENERAL INFORMATION:

St. Martinus University Faculty of Medicine (SMUFOM) originally founded the medical school in 2000 but the university can trace it roots back to 1842 on the island. SMUFOM strives to provide economical medical education that is inspired by excellence. The institution focuses on interdisciplinary study and limits the class size to 60 students each year allowing for a personalized approach to learning. Students are exposed early to the clinical setting starting during the first semester.

The curriculum is modeled after the United States educational system with a strong European influence. SMUFOM is one of only two private medical schools in the Caribbean that offer a two-semester program per year. A traditional four-year medical program and a five and a half-year pre-medical program for motivated high school students are in place. The Pre-Medical Program guarantees acceptance into the medical program after the prerequisite coarse work is successfully completed. SMUFOM believes that to be a competitive residency applicant that students should have actively participated in research. The school sponsors research activities that students are required to participate in either as research assistants or by directing their own project. The school offers student services and study skills enhancements for students in need.

A new 20 acre campus has been built and has modern classrooms, laboratories, instructional facilities, and a library. On-campus housing is available with prices ranging from $450-$600 USD per month depending on occupancy and amenities. Off-campus housing is also available and recommended for married students and students with children. A dress code for students is required.

SMUFOM has an affiliation with the Universidade De Ribeirao Preto (UNAERP) which allows for the exchange of professors and students, and partnerships and collaboration across the educational continuum. No application deadline is in place as the school operates under a rolling admissions system with classes starting in January and July each year. Transfer students are considered but may be required to take a comprehensive entrance examination to determine the appropriate placement.

St. Martinus is not currently credentialed by the American Medical Residency Certification Board (AMRCB®). SMUFOM is listed by the International Medical Education Directory (IMED), the World Health Organization (WHO), and the Medical Council of Canada (MCC). Students are eligible for ECFMG® certification. SMUFOM is chartered by the Government of the Netherlands Antilles Ministry of Education in Curacao.

CURRICULUM:

Pre-Medical program (5 ½ years)

St. Martinus offers an intensive three semester curriculum. Upon successful completion, students will be automatically advanced into the medical program. The pre-medical program is conducted on the St. Martinus campus or in Toronto, Canada in cooperation with CDI College.

Pre Medical Curriculum

Semester I	Semester II	Semester III
Biology I	Biology II	English Writing
Inorganic Chemistry	Organic Chemistry I	Medical Terminology
Physics I	Physics II	Organic Chemistry II
Mathematics	Intro to Anatomical Sciences	Intro to Psychology

M.D. Program

The curriculum is conducted over a four-year program with two semesters each year which last for 20 weeks each. The Basic Sciences are conducted over the first four semesters with the Clinical Science rotations conducted over 72 weeks during years three and four. USMLE® Board review starts early and continues through the entire Basic Science curriculum. A remediation program is available between every semester as needed for students.

Basic Sciences

The Basic Sciences are conducted over the first four semesters on the Curacao campus.

Basic Science Curriculum

Semester I	Semester II	Semester III	Semester IV
Gross Anatomy	Medical Biochemistry	Microbiology and Immunology	Pathology II
Embryology and Human Development.	Behavioral Science	Pathology I	Pharmacology
Medical Histology	Medical Physiology	Epidemiology, Public Health, and Biostatistics	Medical Ethics and Jurisprudence
Medical and Clinical Genetics	Clinical Neuroscience	Integrated Clinical Medicine III	Integrated Clinical Medicine IV
Integrated Clinical Medicine I	Integrated Clinical Medicine II		

Clinical Sciences

The Clinical Science clerkships are conducted over 72 weeks and take place primarily in the United States. Clerkships are also possible in the Netherlands, Curacao, Canada, India, Europe, and the United Kingdom. Students are able to set up their own clerkships as well if desired.

Clinical Science Curriculum

Required – 48 weeks		Electives – 24 weeks	
Internal Medicine	12 - weeks	Anesthesiology	Dermatology
Surgery	12 - weeks (4 week subspecialty included)	Emergency medicine	Family Medicine
Pediatrics	6 - weeks	Gynecology	Internal Medicine
OB/GYN	6 - weeks	Neurology	Obstetrics
Psychiatry	6 - weeks	Occupational Medicine	Ophthalmology
Primary Care / Family Medicine	6 - weeks	Orthopedic Surgery	many others

Grading

Students are promoted from one semester to the next after passing all courses for that semester. In order to successfully complete the Basic Science component of the degree, a student must have successfully passed all courses with a minimum GPA of 2.0. There is a three week, end of semester remediation for students who fail a course or who want a comprehensive review of the subject material. Students must pass USMLE® Step 1 before entering their clinical clerkships.

Grading Policy:

Grade	Notation
A	≥ 90%
B	≥ 80 – 89.5%
C	≥ 70 – 79.5%
F	≤ 69.5%
I	Incomplete due to missing work
W	Withdrawal from school/class
TCG	Transfer Credit Granted

ENTRANCE REQUIREMENTS:

Pre-Medical Program

Students must be high school graduates. The program is often used for students who do not meet the required GPA to be eligible for entrance into the M.D. Program. Students should demonstrate the potential to complete successfully the pre-medical and M.D. programs. Each applicant is reviewed individually by the Admissions Committee. Students will get credit for college level courses they have completed in other academic institutions. Students who successfully complete the Pre-Medical Program proceed automatically into the medical program.

M.D Program

The minimum requirement for admission is 90 semester hours of college level courses. College work must include the following:

- General Biology or Zoology with lab – one academic year
- General Chemistry with lab – one academic year

- Organic Chemistry with lab – one academic year
- Physics with lab – one academic year
- College level English – one academic year
- College level Mathematics or equivalent – one academic year

A generous exposure to studies in the Arts and Sciences is recommended. Coursework in biochemistry is also recommended. The MCAT® is not required but is recommended for all applicants. Those who have taken the test should submit their scores.

SELECTION FACTORS:

The school has an open admissions system and advanced standing is considered for transfer applicants. Admissions are based upon a holistic approach and not on any one specific criterion. Each applicant is reviewed individually. The personal statement is an important aspect of the application allowing the Admissions Committee to understand why an applicant wants to become a physician. A personal interview is conducted either via telephone, Skype, or in person and is the student's opportunity to offer insight into their application. SMUFOM will scrutinize each applicant's intellect, motivation, ability to set priorities and accept responsibility, and overall character traits. Prior medical experience with volunteer work or employment is viewed positively.

Applicants will be notified within two to three weeks of their acceptance status. There is no application deadline as the school operates under a rolling admissions system with classes starting in January and July. A short semester also starts in September and is designed to resolve deficiencies for students who desire to start classes in January or July.

TUITION AND FINANCIAL AID:

Application Fee: $75 USD (non-refundable)

Admission Fee: $1000 USD (non-refundable)

Tuition for Pre-Medical Program (3 semesters): $5,400 USD per semester

Tuition for Basic Sciences (4 semesters): $7,200 USD per semester

Tuition for Clinical Sciences (4 semesters): $12,500 USD per semester

Student Government Fee: $40 USD per semester

Other fees such as laboratory, student, administrative, and graduation may apply.

Several merit based scholarships, awards, and private loans are available. Loans are available for American, Canadian, Indian, and other international students. United States Federal student loans are not available at this time.

No immigration fee is in place for the island, although a refundable deposit of $571-$3143 USD depending on the country of citizenship is required.

ooooo

CURACAO INFORMATION

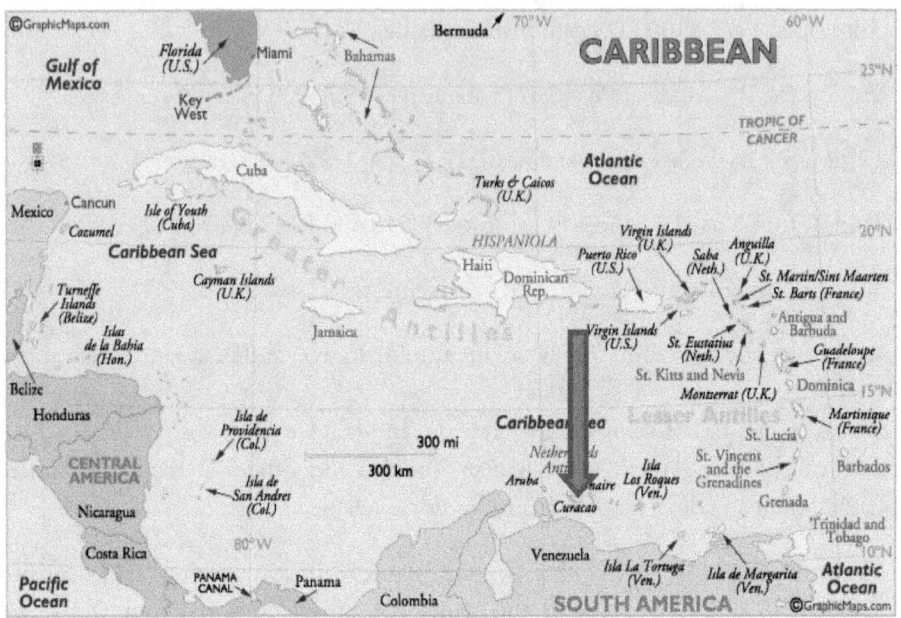

Curacao is an island nation that lies off the coast of Venezuela. Curacao constitutes an area of 171 square miles (444 km^2) and the highest point on the island is Sing Christoffelber at 1,230 ft. (375 m). The uninhabited island of Klein Curacao lies 6.2 miles (10 km) off the southeast coast. Willemstad is the capitol and largest city with the total population of the island at 153,000. The AUSOM, CMU, and St. Martinus campuses are all located in Willemstad.

Curacao is a sovereign state in the Kingdom of the Netherlands operating under a unitary parliamentary representative democracy under a constitutional monarchy. Curacao is one of the former five island territories of the former Netherlands Antilles although the Kingdom of the Netherlands is still responsible for the defense of the island. The island was first contacted by the Spanish in the 1600's and changed hands many times among the Spanish, British, French, and Dutch. These cultures have all influenced the island as has the close proximity to South America.

Profitable industries began with salt mining and have included oil drilling and refining. Currently tourism, international trade, and international financial services are the most important sectors of the economy. The Netherlands Antillean Guilder (ANG) is the official monetary unit of Curacao at an exchange rate of 1 USD to 1.75 ANG. U.S dollars are, however, widely accepted at most locations on the island. Public education is based on the Dutch system.

Curacao has three official languages which are Dutch, English, and Papiamentu. Dutch is the sole language used for all administrative and legal matters. The most widely spoken language is Papiamentu which is a Creole language spoken at all levels of society. Spanish is frequently heard as well. The majority of the citizens self-identify as having African heritage although many races are represented. The majority of inhabitants identify as Roman Catholic at 85% although Christian denominations, Hindu, Muslim, and other religions can be found in small numbers. Curacao also has a thriving Jewish community and has the oldest active Jewish congregation in the Americas dating back to 1651.

The weather is a tropical savannah climate with a dry season from January to September and a wet season from October to December. Temperatures remain relatively constant throughout the year with trade winds keeping the climate comfortable. The coldest month is January with an average temperature of 80°F (27°C) and the warmest month is September with an average temperature is 84°F (29°C). Curacao lies outside of the hurricane belt, and although it has not been impacted directly in over 50 years, the island is typically impacted by pre-hurricane tropical storms. Average rainfall is 21.8 inches (554 mm) per year.

Driving is on the right hand side of the road which is the same as in North America. The time zone is Atlantic Standard Time which is one-hour later than Eastern Standard Time. Electricity is 127/120 volts with 50 cycles which means that most appliances from the United States will work and do not require adapters.

The airport is the Hato International Airport (CUR) located on the northern coast of the island. Hato International Airport was formerly known as the Dr. Albert Plesman International Airport. The airport serves the Caribbean region, South America, North America, and Europe and has the second longest runway in the Caribbean. A new terminal was opened in 2006 and the airport now serves 1.6 million passengers per year.

ooooo

American International School of Medicine

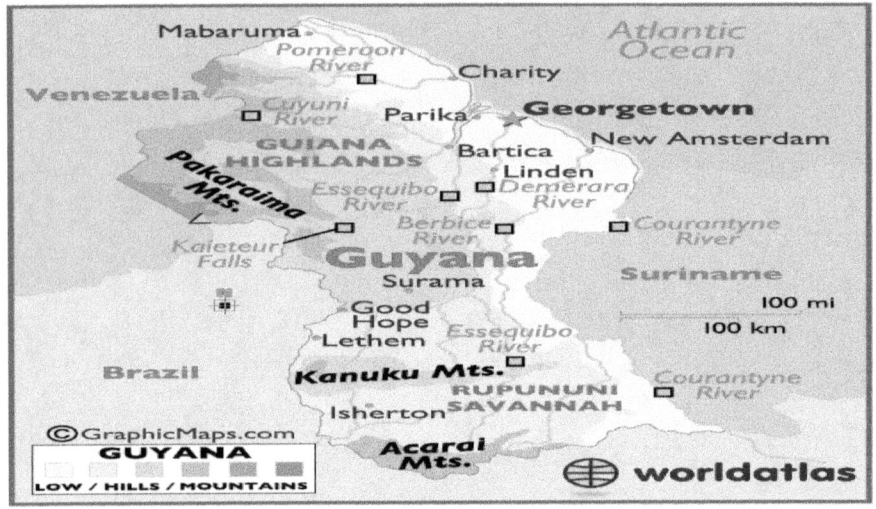

AMRCB® QUICK REFERENCE
American International School of Medicine

Year Founded	1999	Currency	GYD
On-Campus Housing	No	Airport Code	GEO
Pre-Medical Program	Yes	Time Zone	AST (GMT/UTC-4)
MCAT® Required	No	Electricity	240V
Official Language	English	Driving Side	Left

American International School of Medicine

Guyana

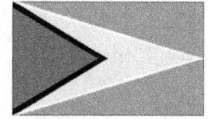

Colin Wilkinson, M.D., Ph.D. – President
Dr. S. Ovid Isaacs – Vice President of Faculty Affairs

CONTACT INFORMATION:

U.S. Admissions Office
American International School
of Medicine
1755 East Park Place Blvd.
Stone Mountain, GA 30086 U.S.A.
Telephone: (404) 756-6737
Toll free: 866-465-9966

Campus Address
American International School
of Medicine
89 Middleton and Sandy Babb Streets, Kitty
Georgetown, Guyana - South America
Telephone: (592) 255-2242
Fax: +1 (413) 674-7301

Canadian Admissions Office
American International School of Medicine
Box 22545 Southbrook Post
Edmonton, AB T6W 0C3

General Information
Website: www.aism.edu/
E-Mail: info@aism.edu
Telephone: (780) 669-7377

GENERAL INFORMATION:

The American International School of Medicine (AISM) was founded in 1999 and began instruction in 2000. Over 380 physicians have graduated from AISM. AISM desires to provide the medical education and training needed to meet the growing demands of healthcare professionals. The school desires to facilitate research and to develop the most advanced and comprehensive education possible. The current USMLE® pass rate is 85%.

The curriculum is modeled after United States medical schools and spans five years. The curriculum is designed to meet regional and international needs. A Pre-Medical program is available for students who have not yet completed the required prerequisites. Modern teaching methods are used and evaluated frequently for effectiveness. AISM offers a Master's of Public Health (M.P.H.) that students can enroll in after completion of their Basic Science rotations.

The main campus is in Georgetown, Guyana with additional training sites in Guyana, the United States, Canada, and England. The Guyana campus utilizes the latest educational technology and included a full library and internet access. No on-campus housing is currently available. AISM has a housing director to aid students in securing housing. No admissions deadline is in place as the school operates under a rolling admissions system with classes starting in January, May, and September each year.

AISM is not currently certified by the American Medical Residency Certification Board (AMRCB®). AISM is listed by the International Medical Education Directory (IMED) and the World Health Organization (WHO). AISM is registered with the National Accreditation Council of Guyana and recognized by the government of Guyana. The Medical Council of India recognizes AISM. Students are eligible for ECFMG® certification.

CURRICULUM:

Pre-Medical Program

The pre-medical program is designed to meet the individual needs of students and is located on the Georgetown, Guyana campus. The program can range from six months to two years depending upon individual needs. Students with no undergraduate credits will need to complete the entire two-year program. Students who have completed the Pre-Medical program and passed the Pre-Medical Comprehensive examinations are promoted into the first year the M.D. program.

Pre-Medical Curriculum

Pre-Med Semester I	Pre-Med Semester II	Pre-Med Semester III
Biology I	Mathematics - Algebra	Intro to Anatomy and Physiology
Chemistry I	Intro to Public Health	Organic Chemistry
Physics I	Intro to Psychology	First Aid Responders
Intro to Medicine	Intro to Epidemiology and Statistics	Nutrition
Verbal Reasoning		Research Paper
Medical History		

M.D. Program

The curriculum is conducted over a four-year program and can be completed in as little as 40 months. The Basic Sciences are conducted over the five semesters followed by six and a half semesters of the Clinical Sciences. Emphasis is placed on academic concentrations, individual opportunities, and the solidification of doctor-patient interviews. Patient exposure begins early in the curriculum.

Basic Sciences

The Basic Sciences are conducted over five semesters which span from 14 to 16 weeks on the campus in Georgetown, Guyana. A comprehensive six-week USMLE® Step I review program takes place in either Atlanta, Georgia U.S.A. or in Guyana.

Basic Science Curriculum

Semester I	Semester II	Semester III	Semester IV	Semester V
Gross Development and Anatomy	Medical Physiology I	Medical Physiology II	Intro to Clinical Medicine I	Intro to Clinical Medicine I (continued)
Histology and Cell Biology	Neurosciences	Medial Microbiology	Pharmacology I	Pharmacology II
Biochemistry and Molecular Biology	Immunology	Behavioral Science	Pathology I	Pathology II
Medical Genetics	Intro to Medicine II	Intro to Medicine III		USMLE® Step I Review
Intro to Medicine I				

Clinical Sciences

The Clinical clerkships are conducted over six and a half semesters divided into 12-week sessions spanning 78 weeks. Clinical rotations are offered in the United States, Canada, the Caribbean, London, United Kingdom, Guyana, and other locations.

Clinical Science Curriculum

Required – 56 weeks		Electives – 22 weeks	
Internal Medicine	12 - weeks	Vascular Surgery	Nephrology
Surgery	12 - weeks	Tropical Medicine	Infectious Disease
Pediatrics	8 - weeks	Urology	Cardiology
OB/GYN	8 - weeks	Sports Medicine	Oncology
Psychiatry	8 - weeks	Radiology	ENT
Family Medicine	8 - weeks	Pulmonary	Many others

Grading

Passing scores range from 75-100%. Examinations are given in USMLE® format in both writing and via computer. Students are promoted from one semester to the next after passing all courses for that semester and achieve graduation after satisfactorily meeting all performance standards. To be eligible for graduation, all students must pass the AISM Clinical Science Comprehensive Examination.

ENTRANCE REQUIREMENTS:

Pre-Medical Program

The program is ideal for students seeking to enter the M.D. track who have not yet completed the required prerequisite coursework. Students who have applied but do meet the standards of admission into the M.D. program may enroll in the Pre-Medical Program to help them qualify. Applicants should have a strong SAT score and strong passes in GCE/CXC/CAPE, or any other advanced level coursework. High scores in English, Mathematics, and the Sciences are expected. Applications are evaluated on a rolling basis.

M.D. Program

The minimum requirement for admission is a baccalaureate degree or the equivalent. Baccalaureate degrees should be in Biology, Chemistry, or one of the associated Sciences. Alternatively, students must have completed and passed a recognized Pre-Medical Program. If applicable, students are required to have six Caribbean Advance Proficiency Examination (CAPE) units including Biology and Chemistry.

The MCAT® is optional but recommended.

SELECTION FACTORS:

AISM has an open admissions policy for students of all backgrounds and seeks to identify applicants who take the medical profession seriously and who have the ability to excel in the program. Students are selected based on their interview, prior academic and life achievements, and their academic skills. Two letters of recommendation are required from college professors or advisors. Official MCAT® scores are optional but recommended. TOEFL® scores are required for students whose native language is not English. The school has an open admissions system and advanced standing is considered for transfer applicants. Applicants will be notified at the earliest possible date of an admissions decision. There is no application deadline as the school operates under a rolling admission system with classes starting in January, May, and September each year.

TUITION AND FINANCIAL AID:

Application Fee: $100 USD (non-refundable)

Tuition for Pre-Medical Sciences:

- -$4,500 USD per semester – International Students
- -$3,500 USD per semester – Guyanese and CARICOM Students

Tuition for Basic Sciences (semesters 1-5):

- -$7,000 USD per semester – International Students
- -$5,000 USD per semester – Guyanese and CARICOM Students

Tuition for Clinical Sciences (semesters 6-11.5):

- -$8,000 USD per semester – International Student
- -$6,000 USD per semester – Guyanese and CARICOM Students

Graduation Fee: $50 USD

Other fees such as laboratory, student, administrative, and transportation may apply.

Several scholarships including merit based and geographic are available. Private loans may be available from outside sources. United States Federal student loans are not available at this time. Students from CARICOM countries are eligible for the CARICOM M.D. Award.

ooooo

Central and South American Medical Schools - Caribbean Region

GreenHeart Medical University School of Medicine

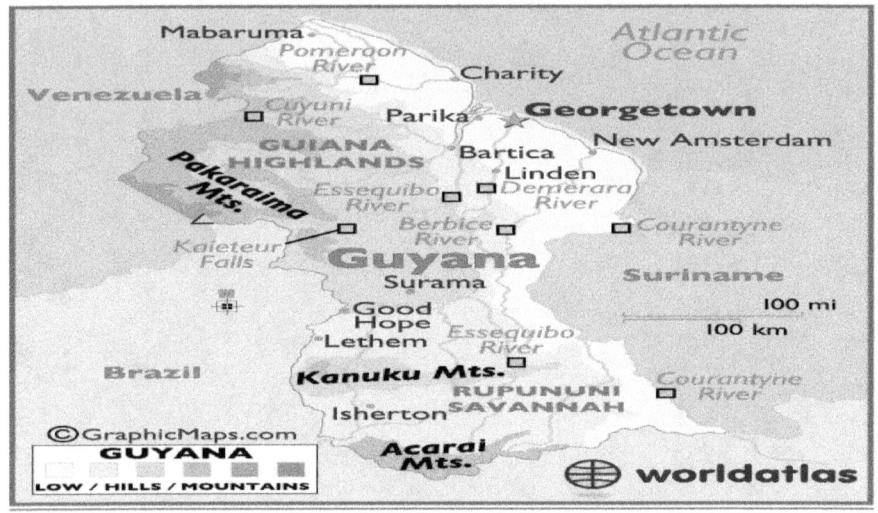

AMRCB® QUICK REFERENCE			
GreenHeart Medical University School of Medicine			
Year Founded	2005	Currency	GYD
On-Campus Housing	No	Airport Code	GEO
Pre-Medical Program	Yes	Time Zone	AST (GMT/UTC-4)
MCAT® Required	No	Electricity	240 V
Official Language	English	Driving Side	Left

GreenHeart Medical University School of Medicine
Guyana

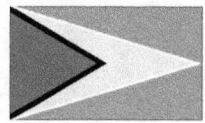

Wayne Barrow – V.P. of Operations

CONTACT INFORMATION:

U.S. Admissions Office
GreenHeart Medical University SOM
Registrar
North American Representative Office
1009 University BLVD. East, NO 201
Silver Spring, MD 20903 U.S.A.
Telephone: 1-855-5-GMU-EDU
Fax: +1 (410) 648-2000

Campus Address
GreenHeart Medical University SOM
#69 Croal Street
Stabroek, Georgetown
Guyana
Telephone: (592) 227-5619
Fax: (592) 225-5612

General Information
Website: http://www.greenheartmed.org/
E-Mail: info@greenheartuniversity.com

GENERAL INFORMATION:

The GreenHeart Medical University School of Medicine (GMU) was founded in 2004 with instruction beginning in 2005. The institution is dedicated to educational innovation, the promotion of ethical values in students, and academic excellence. Students are offered the opportunity to develop the necessary scientific thinking needed to achieve the ability to master the necessary knowledge required of effective physicians. GMU seeks to promote excellence in medical education, research, and health care by training primary health care professionals. Small class sizes are utilized to allow one-on-one interactions between students and faculty.

The curriculum is modeled after United States medical schools and both a four-year and five-year curricula are in place. The school utilizes an integrated curricular approach regarding the practice and theory of medicine as well as clinical exposure. The curriculum aims at facilitating self-directed and self-motivated learning. New teaching and learning methodologies are utilized which include technology. A Pre-Medical Program, Post-Baccalaureate, and a Dual B.S / M.D. degree are both offered. GMU offers programs in nursing and pharmacy as well.

The campus has modern classrooms and utilizes the latest audiovisual equipment. A video library, anatomical models, cadavers, and computers are all available. No on-campus housing is currently available. No admissions deadline is in place as the school operates under a rolling admissions system with classes starting in January, May, and September each year.

GMU is not currently certified by the American Medical Residency Certification Board (AMRCB®). GMU is listed by the International Medical Education Directory (IMED) and the World Health Organization (WHO). GMU is chartered and accredited by the Government of Guyana. Students are eligible for ECFMG® certification.

CURRICULUM:

Pre-Medical Program

The Pre-Medical Program is conducted over two academic years spanning 16 months allowing students to complete all the necessary prerequisite coursework needed for acceptance. Internationally acceptable prerequisite courses are offered and students are allowed flexibility to pursue research and advanced degrees if desired. A Post-Baccalaureate Program is also offered for qualified candidates who do not have sufficient undergraduate or graduate level course and for those desiring to change careers and enter the field of medicine. The Post-Baccalaureate Program offers a customized course structure in less than four semesters. Upon completion of either program, students can directly apply to the GMU M.D. program.

Pre-Medical Curriculum

Pre-Med Semester I	Pre-Med Semester II	Pre-Med Semester III	Pre-Med Semester IV
General Biology I	General Biology II	Intro to Anatomy and Physiology	Intro to Biochemistry
Inorganic Chemistry	Organic Chemistry I	Organic Chemistry II	Research Methodology
College Physics I	College Physics II	Bio-Physics	Medical Ethics
English I	English II	General and Developmental Psychology	Intro to Cellular Biology and Histology
Mathematics I	Mathematics II	Medical Terminology	History and Culture of Guyana

Dual-Degree Program:

A Dual B.S. / M.D. degree program is available for pre-medical students who have not completed a degree and wish to obtain one. The Dual-Degree Program is offered over five years and can be completed in 56 months. Students must enroll initially in the Pre-Medical Program. The program is dived over four semesters of Pre-Medical studies and four semesters of Basic Science study. Students are required to maintain a GPA of 2.5 or higher and take a comprehensive examination before being awarded the Bachelor's in Medical Sciences.

Central and South American Medical Schools - Caribbean Region

Dual B.S. / M.D. Degree

Academic Year I	Academic Year II	Academic Year III	Academic Year IV
General Biology I and II	Intro to Anatomy and Physiology	Anatomy I and II	Neuro-anatomy
Inorganic Chemistry	Organic Chemistry II	Histology	Physiology II
College Physics I and II	Intro to Biochemistry	Embryology	Pathology I and II
English I and II	Research Methodology	Biochemistry I and II	Microbiology
Organic Chemistry I	Medical Terminology	Behavioral Sciences	Medical Research and Bioethics
Mathematics I and II	Bio-Physics	Physiology I	Preventive Medicine
	General and Developmental Psychology	Genetics	Immunology
	Intro to Cellular Biology and Histology	Epidemiology and Public Health	Pharmacology and Therapeutics
	Medical Ethics		Nutrition
	History and Culture of Guyana		

M.D. Program

The curriculum is conducted over a four-year program spanning 40 months. The Basic Sciences are conducted over the first five semesters followed by five semesters of the Clinical Science rotations. Educational methods include lectures, small group seminars, standardized patients, and problem-based workshops. Clinical exposure begins early with longitudinal clinical care experiences.

Basic Sciences

The Basic Sciences are conducted over five semesters on the campus in Georgetown, Guyana.

Basic Science Curriculum

Semester I	Semester II	Semester III	Semester IV	Semester V
Biochemistry I	Anatomy II	Pathology I	Pathology II	Pathophysiology
Histology	Physiology I	Microbiology	Pharmacology and Therapeutics	Physical Diagnosis
Embryology	Biochemistry II	Physiology II	Preventive Medicine	Intro to Clinical Medicine
Anatomy I	Genetics	Neuro-Anatomy	Immunology	Integrated Basic Medical Review
Behavioral Sciences	Epidemiology and Public Health	Medical Research and Bioethics	Nutrition	

Clinical Sciences

The Clinical clerkships are conducted over semesters five through ten spanning 80 weeks and occur in Guyana, the United States, Europe, India, and the United Kingdom. Facilities in Guyana are used primarily although qualified candidates are eligible for rotations elsewhere. Clinical Internships are available for qualified graduates at the Georgetown Public Hospital Corporation which is a 600-bed teaching hospital.

Clinical Science Curriculum

Required – 48 weeks		Electives– 32 weeks
Internal Medicine	12 - weeks	Student Choice
Surgery	12 - weeks	
Pediatrics	6 - weeks	
OB/GYN	6 - weeks	
Psychiatry	6 - weeks	
Family Medicine	6 - weeks	

Grading

Students are promoted from one semester to the next after passing all courses for that semester and achieve graduation after satisfactorily meeting all performance standards. Students are evaluated on quantitative and qualitative measurements. The Dean promotes a student into the Clinical Science clerkship program only after completing all of the Basic Science program requirements and passing the

Comprehensive Examinations. Students must maintain a GPA of 2.0 or greater in the Basic Sciences. The grading system is as follows:

A	between 90-100 points	
B	Between 80-90 points	
C	Between 70-80 points	
D	Between 60-70 points (failing)	
F	Between 50-60 points (failing)	

ENTRANCE REQUIREMENTS:

Pre-Medical Program

The program is ideal for students seeking to enter the M.D. track directly from high school. Students applying for the 5-year program much have competed 12 years of elementary and secondary education or the equivalent. If applicable, students must also have adequate CAPE, GCE 'A' level scores, and CSEC scores.

M.D. Program

The minimum requirement for admission is 90 semester hours of college level courses. A baccalaureate degree or equivalent is preferred and preference will be given to applicants who will have completed this prior to matriculation. College work must include the following (the successful completion of labs are expected with science courses nearly universally even when not specifically listed):

- General Biology – one academic year
- Inorganic Chemistry – one academic year
- Organic Chemistry – one academic year
- Physics – one academic year
- English – one academic year
- Mathematics – one academic year

Courses in Social Sciences and Humanities are desirable. The MCAT® is not required.

SELECTION FACTORS:

The school has an open admissions system and advanced standing is considered for transfer applicants. National and international students are sought that are highly qualified and that come from a diverse background. Students are sought from all segments of society with the goal of creating an ethnic and culturally diverse campus. Passionate and qualified applicants are sought. Applicants are selected based on intellectual curiosity, academic strength, background, and the capacity for learning. Selection is limited to highly qualified students to allow for the best education possible. The personal statement should provide a clear overview of the applicant's personal and academic experience as well as explain the commitment to study at GMU. The Admission Committee seeks to understand the professional and educational goals of the applicant. Two letters of recommendation are required. Students are expected to have minimum undergraduate grades in the prerequisite coursework of a 'C' or higher. Students who are applying from outside of the United States, the United Kingdom,

Canada, or the CARICOM region must submit course-by-course description of their undergraduate coursework. TEOFL® scores must be a minimum of 500 on the paper-based format or 85 on the Internet-based test with a "2" in each section. Academic and non-academic qualifications are both evaluated. Students are evaluated in totality by the Admissions Committee and are invited for an interview if qualified. There is no application deadline as the school operates under a rolling admission system with classes starting in January, May, and September each year.

TUITION AND FINANCIAL AID:

Application Fee: $75 USD (non-refundable)

Payment required to secure acceptance: $1000 USD (non-refundable)

Registration Fee: $500 USD

Enrollment Fee: $150 USD

Kaplan Review: $500-2000 USD

Exit Examination Fee: $500 USD per examination

Graduation Fee: $300 USD

Other fees such as laboratory, student, and administrative may apply.

National (Guyanese) Students:

Tuition for Pre-Medical Sciences (4 semesters): $1,500 USD per semester

Tuition for Basic Sciences (5 semesters): $2,000 USD per semester

Tuition for Clinical Sciences (5 semesters): $2,100 Medicine USD per semester

International Students:

Tuition for Pre-Medical Sciences (4 semesters): $4,550 USD per semester

Tuition for Basic Sciences (5 semesters): $4,900 USD per semester

Tuition for Clinical Sciences (5 semesters): Guyana - $7,000 USD per semester

Tuition for Clinical Sciences (5 semesters): U.S. - $7,000 USD per semester

A limited number of scholarships and student loans are available. Private loans may be available from outside sources. A tuition fee installment and payment plan is available. GMU seeks sponsors for qualified applicants to offset the course of the education. United States federal student loans are not available at this time.

ooooo

Texila American University College of Medicine

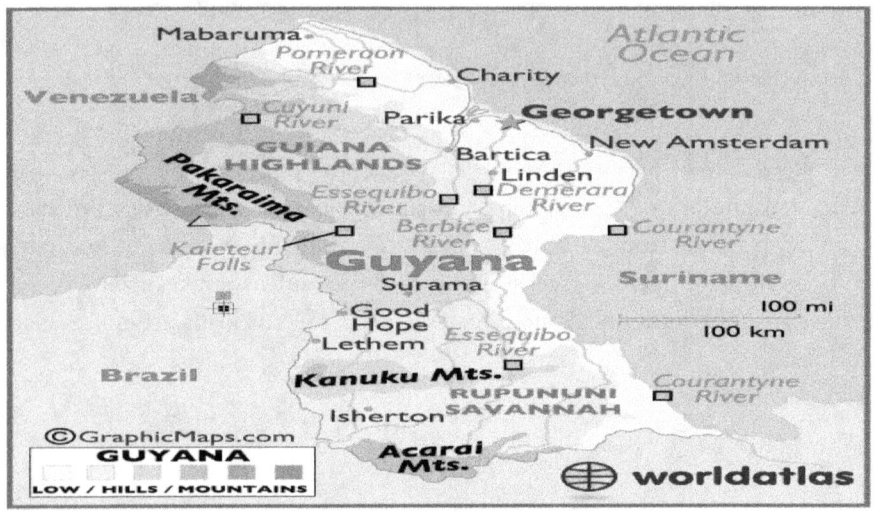

AMRCB® QUICK REFERENCE

Texila American University College of Medicine

Year Founded	2011	Currency	GYD
On-Campus Housing	Yes	Airport Code	GEO
Pre-Medical Program	Yes	Time Zone	AST (GMT/UTC-4)
MCAT® Required	No	Electricity	240 V
Official Language	English	Driving Side	Left

Texila American University College of Medicine

Guyana

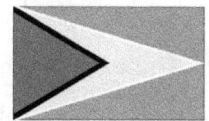

S.P. Saju Bhaskar – President and Chief Executive Officer
Chitra Lakshmi – Vice President
Dr. P.S. Jain – Chancellor

CONTACT INFORMATION:

U.S. Admissions Office
Texila Education Management Services
517 U.S. Highway 1 South, Suite 1190
Iselin, New Jersey 08830 U.S.A.
Telephone: (866) 780-0079
Fax: (855) 528-1230

Campus Address
Texila American University
Lot A, Goedverwagting, Sparendam
East Coast Demerara, Guyana S.A.
Telephone: (+592) 222-5224 / +592
Fax: (+592) 231-8111

Indian Admissions Office
Texila American University
c/o SAKISHI Education Consulting
and Training Limited, #34/1
K.S. Arunachalam Road, K.K. Pudur
Coimbatore-641038 Tamil Nadu, India
Telephone: +91-422-4559900
Fax: +91-422-4559914

Sharjah Admissions Office
Texila American University
TAU Global Consulting Services
c/o India Trade & Exhibition Centere
Office No. 203
P.O Box 66301, Sharjah
United Arab Emirates
Telephone: +9716 5939568

General Information
Website: http://www.tauedu.org/
E-Mail: info@tauedu.org

GENERAL INFORMATION:

The Texila American University (TAU) was founded in 2011 with classes starting in 2011. TAU seeks to build a team from diverse backgrounds and to serve the national and international community. Innovative programs are sought to provide the highest standard of medical training possible and to inspire graduates with humanity and the desire to provide high quality care.

The curriculum is modeled after United States medical schools. A four-year and a five and half-year M.D. program are both available. Students can choose to train in Guyana or in a combination of Guyana and the U.S. A Pre-Medical program is available for students who have not yet completed the required prerequisites. TAU offers combined degrees to include a M.D./M.S., a Masters in Medical Sciences (MMSc) and a research based Ph.D., as well as other degrees in nursing and dentistry as well as distance and on-line programs in behavioral science, clinical research, public health, management, education, and information technology. TAU has partnerships with multiple international institutions including Concordia College in New York where a combined 6-year B.S./M.D. degree is available.

The campus is designed to provide high quality classrooms to generate critical thinking. The infrastructure includes a computer lab, high-tech laboratories, a library, projectors, conference halls, an auditorium, and recreational centers. On-campus housing is guaranteed for all students with housing costs varying per occupancy. No admissions deadline is in place as the school operates under a rolling admissions system with three classes starting each year in January, May, and September.

TAU is not currently certified by the American Medical Residency Certification Board (AMRCB®). TAU is listed by the International Medical Education Directory (IMED) and the World Health Organization (WHO). TAU is accredited by the Accreditation Council of Guyana and recognized by the Medical Council of India. Students are eligible for ECFMG® certification.

CURRICULUM:

Pre-Medical Program – 5.5 years

The Pre-Medical program emphasizing training in the required science subjects and English is conducted over eighteen months spanning four semesters. The instruction takes place on the TAU campus in Guyana. Upon completion, students can directly apply to the TAU M.D. program. Students can pursue the pre-clinical track either on the Guyana campus or in the United States. Students generally complete the first 12 months in their home country and transfer credits directly to TAU. The curriculum consists of four semesters of 16 weeks each.

Participating Universities include the following:

- Broward College, USA
- Charles University, Czech Republic
- Concordia College, USA
- Semmelweis University, Hungary
- Szent Istvan University, Hungary
- University of Debrecen, Hungary
- University of Pecs Medical School, Hungary
- University of Szeged, Hungary
- University of West England (UWE), United Kingdom
- Zamosc University, Poland

Pre-Medical Curriculum

Pre-Med Semester I	Pre-Med Semester II	Pre-Med Semester III	Pre-Med Semester IV
General Biology I	General Biology II	Intro to Histology and Cell Biology	Intro to Anatomy and Physiology
General Chemistry I	General Chemistry II	Organic Chemistry I	Organic Chemistry II
Pre-Calculus	Calculus	General Physics I	Ethics
English I	English II	Psychology	Medical Terminology

M.D. Program

The curriculum is conducted over a four-year program. The Basic Sciences are conducted over the first four semesters, with a fifth "bridge" semester in place which transitions students into the five Clinical Science rotations. The curriculum is designed to reinforce the tenets of medicine.

Basic Sciences

The Basic Sciences are conducted over four, 16-week semesters on the campus in Guyana. The fifth semester is designed to transition into clinical medicine and to prepare students for USMLE® Step 1. The fifth semester takes place over 16 weeks.

Basic Science Curriculum

Semester I	Semester II	Semester III	Semester IV
Medical Embryology	Behavioral Sciences	Pathology I	Pathology II
Biostatistics and Epidemiology	Medical Biochemistry	Medical Microbiology	Pharmacology
Gross Anatomy	Medical Physiology	Medical Ethics	Community Medicine Preventive
Histology, Cell, and Molecular Biology	Genetics	Medical Parasitology	Forensic Medicine and Toxicology
Medical Genetics	Evidence Based Medicine and Research	Immunology	Integrative Medicine II
Health Corps	Research Writing	Health Corps	Health Corps
	Health Corps	Integrated Clinical Medicine I	
	Neuroscience	Health Corps	

Clinical Sciences

The Clinical clerkships are conducted over semesters six through ten over 80 weeks and occur in United States and other locations. TAU has an affiliation with the Georgetown Public Hospital Cooperation. U.S. placements currently occur in Georgia, Maryland, and Illinois.

Clinical Science Curriculum

Required – 48 weeks		Electives– 32 weeks	
Internal Medicine	12 - weeks	Radiology	Dermatology
Surgery	12 - weeks	Anesthesia	Dentistry
Pediatrics	6 - weeks	Orthopedics	ENT
OB/GYN	6 - weeks	Emergency	Cardiology
Psychiatry	6 - weeks	Critical Care	Ophthalmology
Orthopedics	6 - weeks	Pulmonology	many others

Grading

Students are promoted from one semester to the next after passing all courses for that semester and achieve graduation after satisfactorily meeting all performance standards. The Dean promotes a student into the Clinical Science clerkship program only after completing all of the Basic Science program requirements.

ENTRANCE REQUIREMENTS:

Pre-Medical Program

The program is designed for students seeking to enter the M.D. track directly from high school. Applicants must have completed 10-12 years of high school Students should have passes in Chemistry, Biology, Physics, and Mathematics. Students with 90-credit hours of college credits can enter a focused Basic Science Program.

M.D. Program:

The minimum requirement for admission is 90 semester hours of undergraduate college level courses. The successful completion of a baccalaureate or an associate degree in any relevant science area is required. College work must include the following (the successful completion of labs are expected with science courses nearly universally even when not specifically listed):

- Biology
- General Chemistry
- Organic Chemistry
- Physics
- English
- Calculus

The MCAT® is not required.

SELECTION FACTORS:

The school has an open admissions system and advanced standing is considered for transfer applicants at any semester. AUS receives over one thousand applications per year for the M.D. program. Students can apply prior to all perquisites being completed and applicants are not considered based on citizenship and/or residency. Applicants are expected to have exceeded expectations, to have challenged themselves academically, and to have demonstrated service and commitment to activities. TAU seeks diversity and students who will contribute and enhance the overall learning environment. The prior academic performance and difficulty of academic study is the most important factor in student selection although individual, personal, and academic circumstance is considered. Each student application is reviewed at least twice in its entirety and no set formula is in place to select students. A strong personal statement is expected and an applicant's overall story should be accurately represented. Honors, achievements, personal strengths, future goals, and the prior activities of each student are also considered. Grades are expected to not have declined over time and achievements outside of the classroom that demonstrate personal skills and strengths are sought. Traits such as concern, intellectual curiosity, motivation, generosity, creativity, perseverance, determination, and demonstrated leadership ability are desired. Letters of recommendation should be from persons who can discuss the applicant's character, accomplishments, and capabilities although additional letters of support are accepted also from persons who know the student well. Applicants will be notified within days to weeks of their acceptance status after the application is complete. There is no application deadline as the school operates under a rolling admission system with classes starting in January, May, and September each year.

TUITION AND FINANCIAL AID:

Application Fee: $150 USD (non-refundable)

Registration Fee: $150 USD

Security Deposit: $1,000 (refundable)

Tuition for Pre-Medical Sciences (4 semesters): $4,200 per semester

Tuition for Basic Sciences (4 semesters): $5,400 USD per semester

Tuition for 5th semester: $5,400 USD

Tuition for Clinical Sciences (5 semesters): $6,995 USD per semester

Graduation Fee: $1,000 USD

Other fees such as laboratory, malpractice, student, and administrative may apply.

A number of full and partial scholarships are available and scholarship criteria are competitive. Partial grants are also available for students with GPA's of at least 3.8 or higher. Private loans are available from outside sources and TAU is committed to provide all available financial help to students that is available. A full tuition waiver is available for one Guyanese citizen and one CARICOM student each year. United States Federal student loans are not available at this time.

ooooo

University of Guyana Faculty of Health Sciences

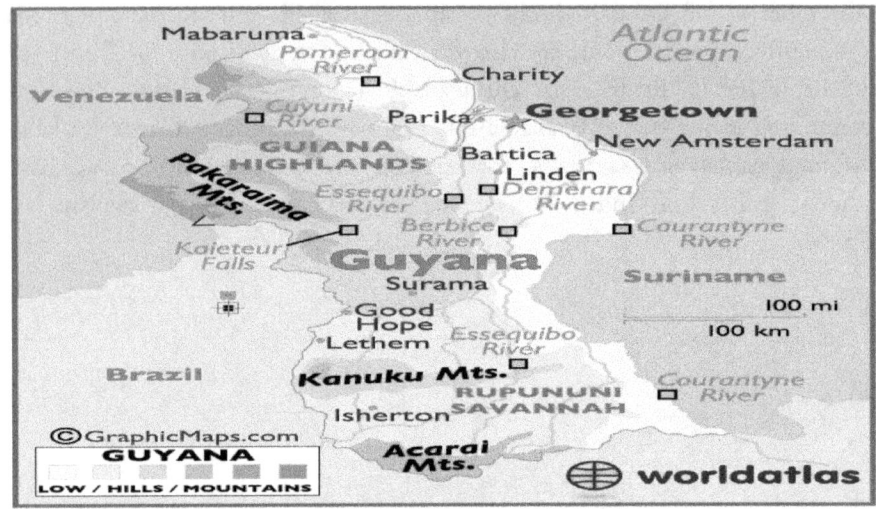

AMRCB® QUICK REFERENCE

University of Guyana Faculty of Health Sciences

Year Founded	1985	Currency	GYD
On-Campus Housing	Yes	Airport Code	GEO
Pre-Medical Program	No	Time Zone	AST (GMT/UTC-4)
MCAT® Required	No	Electricity	240 V
Official Language	English	Driving Side	Left

University of Guyana Faculty of Health Sciences

Guyana

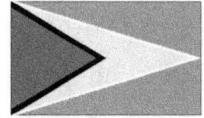

Bertrand Ramcharan – Chancellor
Dr. Madan Rambaran – Director, School of Medicine
Dr. Emanuel Cummings – Dean, Faculty of Health Sciences

CONTACT INFORMATION:

Campus Address
University of Guyana
Turkeyen Campus
P.O. Box 10-1110
Greater Georgetown, Guyana
Telephone: +592 222-5404
Fax: +592 222-3570

General Information
Website: http://uog.edu.gy/faculties/fhs/
E-Mail: publicrelations@uog.edu.gy

GENERAL INFORMATION:

The University of Guyana School of Medicine (UGSM) was found in 1985 with first graduating class in 1991. The parent university in Guyana was established in 1963 and has a current enrollment of over 5000 students. UGSM has graduated over 350 doctors since instruction began. The principle goal of the school is to graduate physicians that are skillful, knowledgeable, and have the behavior and attitude that enables general, community-based practice. The mission of UGSM is to disseminate, generate, discover, and apply knowledge of the highest standard.

The 5-year curriculum is modeled after United States and British educational systems and an M.B.B.S. degree is conferred upon graduation. The curriculum has been adapted over the last 10 years to include problem-based learning and non-cadaveric virtual anatomy teaching. The University strives to keep the curriculum up-to-date. UGSM offers programs in Pharmacy, Public Health, Optometry, and Dentistry as well.

A major physical plant rehabilitation and expansion program has recently been completed allowing for the addition of several new buildings and more classroom space. Three separate student resident halls are available and housing is available for approximately 130 students each year at a cost of $125 USD per month. Admissions take place just once yearly for the class that starts in September. It is recommended that applications be submitted no later than February of the year desired

UGSM is not currently certified by the American Medical Residency Certification Board (AMRCB®). UGSM is listed by the International Medical Education Directory (IMED) and the World Health Organization (WHO). UGSM is accredited by the Accreditation Council of Guyana. UGSM is accredited by the

Caribbean Accreditation Authority for Education in Medicine and other Health Professions (CAAM-HP). Students are eligible for ECFMG® certification.

CURRICULUM:

M.D. Program

The curriculum is conducted over a five-year program and provides an M.B.B.S. degree upon completion. The entire curriculum is conducted over 222 weeks.

Basic Sciences

The Basic Sciences curriculum is conducted over 76 weeks of core pre-clinical study. The curriculum is under review and is not available at the time of this publication. Contact UGSM directly for additional information.

Clinical Sciences

The Clinical clerkships are conducted over 146 weeks. Clerkships are conducted primarily at the Georgetown Public Hospital Corporation in Guyana.

Grading

Students are promoted from one semester to the next after passing all courses for that semester and achieve graduation after satisfactorily meeting all performance standards. The Dean promotes a student into the Clinical Science clerkship program only after completing all of the Basic Science program requirements

ENTRANCE REQUIREMENTS:

M.D. Program

General entry requirements are as follows:

- Applicants must possess at least three subjects at GCE 'A' level with a minimum grade of C or CAPE Unit 1 and 2, with a minimum grade III, in any two of these subjects – Physics, Chemistry, Biology or Mathematics.

Applicants from the North American educational system are expected to have completed the standard science prerequisite coursework necessary for success in medical study which includes the following:

- General Biology or Zoology with labs – one academic year
- Inorganic or General Chemistry with labs – one academic year
- Organic Chemistry with labs – one academic year
- Physics with labs – one academic year
- English – two academic semesters
- Mathematics – one academic year

The MCAT® is not required.

SELECTION FACTORS:

Transfer applicants are considered on an individual basis. Students are selected based on their overall academic ability. Academic ability is judged based on prior grads and educational success. Students are sought that have a sound character and personality consistent with successful graduates. Selected applicants will have demonstrated an aptitude for science and medicine. Letters of recommendation are important as are the personal essay and personal interview. Admissions take place just once yearly for the class that starts in September each year. It is recommended that applications be submitted no later than February of the year desired. Applicants will be notified at the earliest possible date of an admissions decision.

TUITION AND FINANCIAL AID:

Application Fee: $5 USD (non-refundable)

Tuition Categories

- **Guyanese Students**

    Those who are Guyanese either by birth or naturalization AND who have been resident in Guyana for a minimum period of two (2) years prior to the commencement of the relevant academic year are required to pay the current local tuition fee of: $2350 USD per year.

- **Foreign students**

    Foreign students are required to pay annual tuition fees of $6,200 USD per year.

Examination Fees: $60 USD per year

Other fees such as laboratory, library, information technology, student, administrative, and graduation apply.

Private loans may be available from outside sources. United States Federal student loans are not available at this time.

ooooo

Central and South American Medical Schools - Caribbean Region

GUYANA INFORMATION

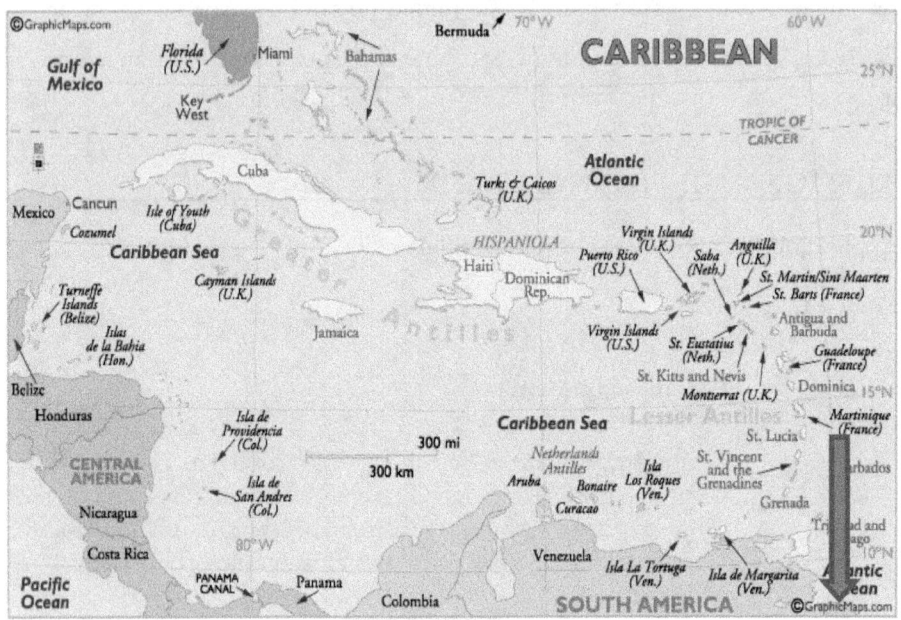

Guyana is located on the South American continent. It is bordered by the Atlantic Ocean to the North, Suriname to the east, Brazil to the South, and Venezuela to the West. The county has one of the largest unspoiled rainforest in South America and over 80% of the country is covered by forest. The highest point in the country is Mount Roraima at 9,219 feet (2,810 m).

Guyana has a total area of 83,000 square miles (214,969 km²) and has 285 miles (459 km) of coastline. Kiaeteur Falls is a major attraction located in Guyana and is five times higher than Niagara Falls. The population is 740,000 persons and it is the 8th least densely population in the world. However, nearly 90% of the population lives in a narrow coastal strip along the Atlantic Ocean. The capital city is Georgetown with a population of 235,000 persons. The Texila Medical University campus is located in East Coast Demerara. The campuses of AISM, the University of Guyana, and GreenHeart are all in Georgetown.

The official name of the country is the Cooperative Republic of Guyana. The government is a unitary semi-presidential republic. Guyana was originally colonized by the Netherlands and later became a British Colony named British Guyana. Guyana gained independence from the United Kingdom in 1966 officially becoming a republic in 1970. Guyana is part of the Common Wealth of Nations and is a member of the Caribbean Community and Common Market (CARICOM). Guyana is also a founding member of the Union of South American Nations.

The official language is English and Guyana is the only English speaking country in South America. Although English is the official language, the national language is Guyanese Creole. Hindustani is widely spoken as well. The culture is similar to other English-speaking Caribbean countries. The population is 43% East Indian origin from descendants of indentured laborers from India, 43% Afro-Guyanese descendants from African slaves, with the remaining populace coming from varying backgrounds. Nearly 60% of the population identifies as Christian, 28% are Hindu, and 7% are Muslims. The only major sport in the country is cricket which is widely popular.

The economy is primarily agricultural with the main crops consisting of sugar and rice. Mining, timber, and fishing are also important to the economy. The currency is the Guyanese dollar (GYD) with an exchange rate of one GYD to 0.0049 USD. The time zone is UTC-4 which is the same as the Atlantic Standard

Time Zone in the United States. Electricity in the county is 240 volts/60 cycles thus an adapter is required for North American appliances.

The climate is tropical and hot and humid although the coast is moderated by northeast trade winds. Seasonal variations are slight. Guyana lies outside of the hurricane belt and no hurricanes have impacted the county over hundreds of years. The average high temperature is 90°F (32°C) with July being the hottest month and February being the coolest. The highest temperature ever recorded in Georgetown was 93°F (34°C) and the lowest 68°F (20°C). The humidity is 70% year-round. The northwest part of the country receives the most rainfall and the southeast interior receives the least. A rainy season exists from May to July and November through January along the coast, and from April through September farther inland. Average rainfall is 98 in (2500 mm) each year.

The only international airport in Guyana is the Cheddi Jagan International Airport (GEO). The airport is located 25 mi (41 km) south of Georgetown and is currently undergoing a $150 million dollar expansion slated to be completed in late 2015. Regional flights are available from Canada, the United States, and other countries. Direct fights are available from Toronto, Miami, Atlanta, and New York. Guyana does have a departure tax of $10.75 USD. Visas are required of all visitors to the country with the exception of the United States, Canada, South Korea, Japan, the European Union, and certain other commonwealth countries. Driving in on the left-hand side of the road which is the opposite of the driving side in North America.

ooooo

Central and South American Medical Schools - Caribbean Region

University of the West Indies Faculty of Medicine - St. Augustine

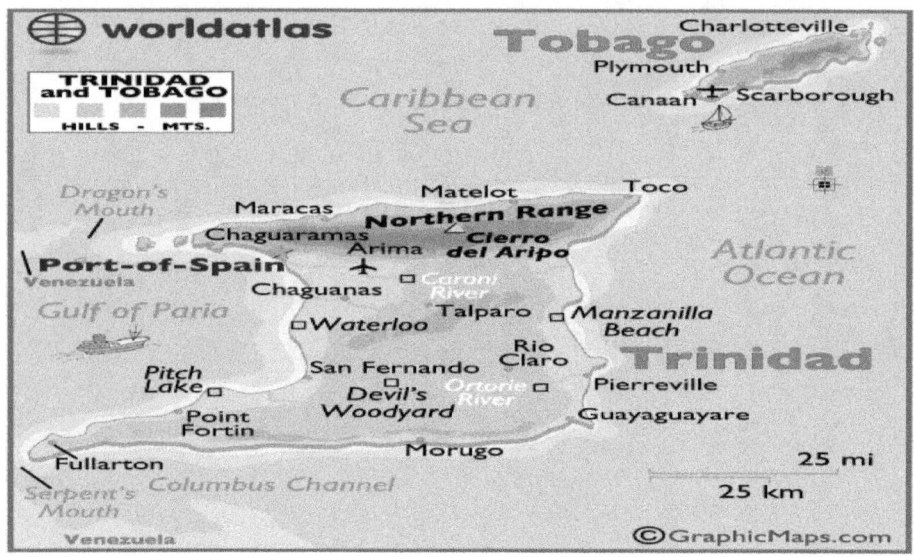

AMRCB® QUICK REFERENCE
University of the West Indies Faculty of Medicine

Year Founded	1989	Currency	TTD
On-Campus Housing	Yes	Airport Code	POS
Pre-Medical Program	Yes	Time Zone	AST (GMT/UTC-4)
MCAT® Required	No	Electricity	115 V / 60 H
Official Language	English	Driving Side	Left

University of the West Indies Faculty of Medicine – St. Augustine

Trinidad and Tobago

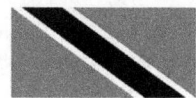

Prof. Samuel Ramsewek – Dean
Dr. Yuri Clement – Deputy Dean of Basic Health Sciences
Dr. Ian Sammy – Deputy Dan of Clinical Sciences

CONTACT INFORMATION:

Campus Address
Office of the Dean
Faculty of Medical Sciences
Eric Williams Medical Science Complex
Building 39, First Floor
Uriah Butler Highway, Champ Fleurs
Trinidad, West Indies

General Information
Telephone: (868) 645-3232 ext 5025-7
Fax: (868) 663-9836
Website: http://sta.uwi.edu/fms/
E-Mail: deanfms@sta.uwi.edu

GENERAL INFORMATION:

The University of the West Indies Faculty of Medicine – St. Augustine (UWI) began physician education in 1989. The University of the West Indies Faculty of Medical Sciences (FMS) began initially in 1948 as an overseas College of the University of London. The first campus of FMS was at the Mona campus in Kingston, Jamaica with another campus in Barbados at Cave Hill in addition to the St. Augustine campus. The University of the West Indies serves as the tertiary educational University for fourteen Caribbean (CARICOM) countries and the total enrollment across all campuses and disciplines is over 40,000 students. The University of the West Indies serves the countries of the Commonwealth Caribbean which include: Anguilla, Antigua/Barbuda, the Bahamas, Barbados, Belize, the British Virgin Islands, Cayman Islands, Dominica, Grenada, Jamaica, Montserrat, St. Christopher-Nevis, St. Lucia, St. Vincent and the Grenadines, Trinidad and Tobago, and the Turks and Caicos Islands. Over 7,000 physicians have graduated from UWI across all campuses.

The mission of the University of the West Indies Faculty of Medicine medical school in Trinidad and Tobago is to recruit and train students to improve the healthcare delivery system by striving for professional excellence throughout their career. The curriculum is a five-year program modeled after the U.S. and British educational systems and offers an M.B.B.S. degree over five years. An M.D. degree is a research degree and specialist qualification takes an additional four years of training and is offered in Anesthesia, General Internal Medicine, Ophthalmology, Orthopedics, Pediatrics, Psychiatry, Radiology, Surgery, and Urology (similar to a medical residency in the United States). A Master of Science in Clinical Psychology is also available. The medical education is offered via problem-based learning involving small-groups and supplemental didactic lectures. Interested students are able to pursue research in the areas of anatomy, biochemistry, physiology, pharmacology, and public health. A Pre-Health Professions Program is available as well to allow applicants to meet the requirements for matriculation.

The medical school campus is housed in the Eric Williams Medical Science Complex. The complex was built in 2002 and is a comprehensive structural environment for multidisciplinary education. The school of nursing, dental, pharmacy, and veterinary medicine are housed here as well as the Mt. Hope Hospital, computer-assisted learning facilities, library, and administrative facilities. On-campus student housing is available.

UWI is listed by the International Medical Education Directory (IMED) and is listed by the World Health Organization (WHO). At the time of this publication, UWI is not currently certified by the American Medical Residency Certification Board (AMRCB®). Students are eligible for ECFMG® certification. UWI is accredited by the Caribbean Accreditation Authority for Medicine and other Health Professions (CAAM-HP).

CURRICULUM:

Pre-Health Professions Program

The program is conducted over three semesters only on the St. Augustine campus. Upon completion, students will have completed all the required prerequisites for the M.B.B.S. program and be offered admission.

Pre-Health Professions Program

Semester I	Semester II	Semester III
Biology I – Intro to Cellular and Molecular	Biology II – Basic Microbiology	Biology III – Mammalian Anatomy and Physiology
Chemistry I – Chemical Fundamentals	Chemistry II – Chemical Principles	Chemistry III – Intro to General Biochemistry
Mathematics I – General Mathematics	Mathematics II – Applied with Statistics I	Mathematics III – Applied with Statistics II
Physics I – Mechanics	Physics II – Electricity, Light, Atomic, and Nuclear Structures	Physics III
English I	English II	

M.D. Program

The curriculum follows the British style of education and is conducted over a five-year program and consists of two phases and ten semesters. Students are required to complete a minimum of nine foundation credits of Foundation Courses prior to starting the Basic Sciences. Phase I consists of the first three year of Basic Science education (five and a half semesters) and Phase II consists of the Clinical Science education (four and a half semesters).

Basic Sciences

The Basic Sciences are conducted over five and a half semesters on the campus on Trinidad and Tobago.

Phase I - Basic Science Curriculum

Year 1	Year 2	Year 3
Environment and Health	Respiration	Applied Para-Clinical Sciences I
Base Para-Clinical Sciences	Neuroscience and Behavior	Applied Para-Clinical Sciences II
Digestion and Metabolism	Endocrine and Reproduction	Applied Para-Clinical Sciences III
Cardiovascular and Renal	Muscles, Bones, and Joints	Integrated Para-Clinical Sciences

Clinical Sciences

The majority of clinical training takes place at the Mt. Hope Hospital in Trinidad.

Phase II - Clinical Science Curriculum

Year 4 – Clinical Rotations (year long)	Year 5 – Clinical Rotations (year long)
Clinical Medicine I	Clinical Medicine II
Child Health I	Child Health II
Community Health I	Community Health II
Psychiatry	Otorhinolaryngology
OB/ GYN I	OB / GYN II
General Surgery I	General Surgery II (Neurosurgery and Pediatric Surgery)
	Ophthalmology
	Anesthesia and Intensive Care
	Orthopedic Surgery

*Electives include:

> Accident and Emergency, Adult Medicine, Anesthesiology, Child Health, Community Health, Dentistry, Emergency Medicine, ENT, Family Medicine, General Medicine, General Surgery, Hematology. Immunology, OB / GYN, Ophthalmology, Orthopedics, Pathology, Radiology, Pediatrics, and Psychiatry

Grading

Students are promoted from one year to the next after passing all courses for that semester and achieve graduation after satisfactorily meeting all performance standards. The Dean promotes a student into the Clinical Science clerkship program only after completing all of the Basic Science program requirements.

Grading Scheme:

80-100: Distinction

75-79: Honors I

70-74: Honors II

50-69: Pass

<50: Fail

ENTRANCE REQUIREMENTS:

Pre-Medical Program

The 35-credit program is available only on the UWI St. Augustine campus. The program starts in August each year and has space for 32 students each year. Students will need to maintain a cumulative Grade Point Average of 3.0. Students earn a certificate at the end of the program. Students who do not meet the requirements for admission into the M.D. program in St. Augustine may be eligible for admission into other UWI Faculty of Medical Science programs. The program is not designed for nationals of Trinidad and Tobago.

Prospective candidates should have the following:

- A minimum grade point average (GPA) of 3.0 in English, Chemistry, Biology, Physics, Mathematics, and a foreign language (Grade 12 matriculation)

OR

- Five 'O' level passes with grades A, B, and C in the same subjects or European equivalents

- Consideration will be given to students transferring from other fields to the health professions.

M.D. Program

The minimum acceptable requirements to the M.B.B.S. program are based on the Caribbean Proficiency (CAPE) Examination. Students are expected to have a degree in the basic sciences and the following:

- Passes in at least five subjects a CXC (CSEC) General Proficiency (Grades I or II and from 1998 Grade III) or GCE O-levels, or approved equivalents which must include English Language, Mathematics, Chemistry, Biology, and Physics

- SCHEME A: Passes in both Units of Chemistry, Biology, and one other subject at CAPE or GCE A-level or approved equivalent; or

- SCHEME B: Passes in Chemistry, Biology/Zoology, and any other subject a N1 (open Campus)

Applicants from the North American educational system will be evaluated on an individual basis. Students with specific majors and GPA's will be given greater consideration for acceptance. All applicants to the University who are not native English speakers must take an English Proficiency Test such as the TOEFL®.

SELECTION FACTORS:

The school does accept inter-facility and inter-campus transfer students from within the UWI educational system. Other transfer students will be considered as well and acceptance will be based on performance in Chemistry, Biology and other subjects. Transfer students must have a minimum GPA of 3.0 in order to be considered. UWI notes that the M.B.B.S. medical program is highly competitive and meeting the qualifications for acceptance does not guarantee acceptance. Students must submit an autobiographical sketch explaining the reasons for their career choice in medicine. Co-curricular activities are expected and certified evidence of involvement should be submitted as well with recent involvement expected. Applicants may be required to attend an interview.

TUITION AND FINANCIAL AID:

The cost of medical education is dependent up the country of residency. Students who belong to a "contributing country" have a lower overall expense than do the citizens of "non-contributing" countries. Contributing countries are Caribbean Community (CARICOM) countries. The University of the West Indies is partially funded by governments of the CARICOM countries that contribute to the yearly budget.

CARICOM members include:

Antigua and Barbuda	Bahamas	Barbados	Belize
Dominica	Grenada	Guyana	Haiti
British Virgin Islands	Montserrat	Suriname	Anguilla
Saint Kitts and Nevis	Saint Lucia	Bermuda	Jamaica Saint
Vincent and the Grenadines		Trinidad and Tobago	

Total tuition for CARICOM contributing countries - sponsored: $4,015 USD per year

Total tuition for CARICOM contributing countries – non-sponsored: $6,691 USD per year

Total tuition for Pan-Caribbean countries - sponsored: $8,364 USD per year

Total tuition for non-contributing countries: $22,288 USD per year

Other fees such as laboratory, student, administrative, and graduation may apply.

Multiple merit based scholarships and private loans are available although primarily for citizens from CARICOM countries. United States Federal student loans are not available at this time.

ooooo

TRINIDAD AND TOBAGO INFORMATION

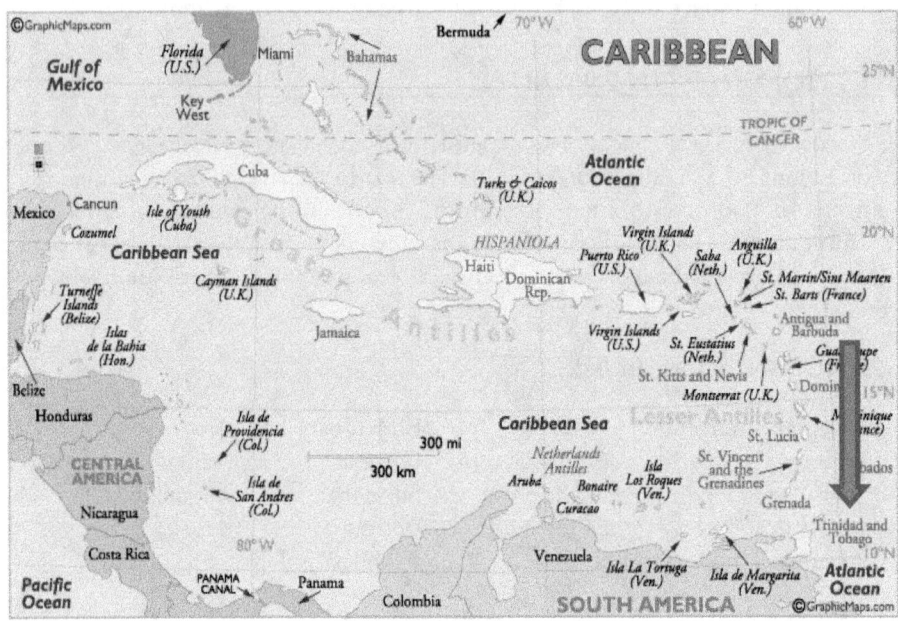

Trinidad and Tobago are the southernmost of the Caribbean islands, located just off the coast of Venezuela and at the Southeasterly tip of the Antilles. Tobago is 20 miles (32 km) to the northeast of Trinidad and has an area of 120 square miles (311 km^2). Trinidad has an area of 1,864 square miles (4828 km^2). The island of Tobago is comprised of a single volcanic mountain and rises to an elevation of 1,804 feet (550 m). Trinidad is comprised of three ranges and the highest point is El Cerro del Aripo at 3,084 feet (940 m). The capital city is the Port-of-Spain with a population of 63,900 persons and the total population of the country is 1.3 million persons. Geographically, the island lies on the continental shelf of South America and is considered to be part of South America. However, the West Indies are generally considered to be part of North America and the langue and cultural links of the islands are primarily linked to North America. The UWI campus is located in Champ Fleurs.

Trinidad, along with Tobago and several smaller islands, officially form the Republic of Trinidad and Tobago which is an independent state in the Commonwealth of Nations. The government is officially a unitary parliamentary constitutional republic. The islands became independent from the United Kingdom in 1962 forming the republic in 1976. The majority of the population lives on Trinidad (96%) and thus Trinidad is the more developed of the two islands while Tobago is more serene. The population primarily consists of peoples of African descent and East Indians. The official language is English and this is the primary language spoken. Spanish, local Creole dialects and Hindi can also be heard. Historically, the islands have been under Spanish, British, Dutch, and French possession. Christianity is the primary religion but Anglicans, Protestants, Hindus, and Muslims also practice on the islands.

The economy is chiefly based on petroleum products which provide citizens with a per capita income significantly above the Latin American average. Tourism and agriculture are also important with sugarcane, coconuts, citrus fruits, rubber trees, and coffee being the important export products. The overall climate is tropical with an average year round temperature on the islands is 85°F (29°C). The dry season spans the first six months of the calendar year followed by the wet season in the second half of the year. The islands are located outside of the hurricane belt.

The unit of currency is the Trinidad and Tobago dollar (TTD) with an exchange rate of 1.0 U.S. dollar to 6.43 TTD's. The time zone is UTC-4 which is the same as the Atlantic Standard Time Zone in the United States. The electricity is 115 V / 60 H thus an adapter is not needed for North American appliances.

Trinidad and Tobago are served by the Piarco International Airport (POS) located in Piarco on the island of Trinidad. Several international airlines and charter companies provide scheduled flights to Trinidad and Tobago. Flights are available from the United States, Canada, Britain, Germany, Venezuela, and other Caribbean countries. Available airlines include Air Canada, Air Jamaica, ALM, American Airlines, British Airways, Caribbean Airlines, Jet Blue, LIAT, and United Airlines. Driving is on the left side of the road which is the opposite of North America.

ooooo

About the Author

I did not decide to become a physician until I was in my late 20's and did not actually apply to medical school until I was 30 years old. At this juncture in my life, I was happily married, had a 6-year-old daughter, and was well into my original career choice, which was as a firefighter and a paramedic. It was not at all easy to return to college full-time while I worked full-time and enjoyed my family. I knew that I wanted to be a physician, however, and was prepared to do what was necessary to accomplish this.

My intention from the beginning was to matriculate into a United States medical school. Knowing that competition was fierce, I was a realist when it came to understanding that it was completely possible that I might not get accepted. It was at this point that I began researching international medical schools and the procedures that would be required to practice medicine in the United States were I to graduate from one of these schools. I quickly discovered that no complete resources existed to provide me with the information that I needed on schools located throughout the Caribbean region. Consequently, this book was born.

I have since graduated from Mercer University School of Medicine in Macon, Georgia U.S.A. I completed a combined residency in Internal Medicine and Psychiatry at Dartmouth in New Hampshire and obtained a Master's Degree in Health Policy from the Dartmouth Institute. I continued to work clinically and hold the position of the Chief Medical Officer at a Dartmouth affiliated hospital. Subsequently, I was asked to lead the American Medical Residency Certification Board® and function as the Chief Executive Officer. I am very thankful for my education and training in the United States; however, I would have gone to the Caribbean without regret for my education had this been necessary. This book will hopefully provide guidance to prospective students so that they, too, can matriculate into the medical school of their choice, whether it is in the Caribbean region or elsewhere.

Steven W. Powell, MD, MPH, CPE, FAPA

References

Information was obtained directly from school representatives, fliers, individual school catalogues, and websites of the following schools:

AMERICAN GLOBAL UNIVERSITY
Website: http://www.agusm.org/

AMERICAN INTERNATIONAL SCHOOL OF MEDICINE
Website: http://www.aism.edu/

AUREUS UNIVERSITY SCHOOL OF MEDICINE
Website: http://www.aureusuniversity.com

AVALON UNIVERSITY SCHOOL OF MEDICINE
Website: http://www.avalonu.org

AVICINA MEDICAL ACADEMY
Website: htto://www.info@avicina.bz

CARIBBEAN MEDICAL UNIVERSITY SCHOOL OF MEDICINE
Web: http://www.cmumed.org

CENTRAL AMERICA HEALTH SCIENCES UNIVERSITY
Website: http://www.cahsu.edu/

COLUMBUS UNIVERSITY SCHOOL OF MEDICINE AND HEALTH SCIENCES
Website: http://2nsc-2010-a.com/

GRACE UNIVERSITY SCHOOL OF MEDICINE
Website: http://www.grace-usom.org/

GREENHEART UNIVERSTIY SCHOOL OF MEDICINE
Website: http://www.greenheartmed.org/

HOPE UNIVERSITY SCHOOL OF MEDICINE
Website: http://www.hopeuniversity.org/

INTERAMERICAN MEDICAL UNIVERSITY
Website: http://www.interamericanschool.com/

MEDICAL UNIVERSITY OF THE AMERICAS
Website: http://www.mua.edu.bz

SAINT JAMES SCHOOL OF MEDICINE – BONAIRE
Website: http://bonaire.sjsm.org/

ST. LUKE'S UNIVERSITY SCHOOL OF MEDICINE
Website: http://www.stluke.edu.bz

ST. MARTINUS UNIVERSITY FACULTY OF MEDICINE
Website: http://www.martinus.edu

ST. MATTHEW'S UNIVERSITY SCHOOL OF MEDICINE
Website: http://www.stmatthews.edu/

TEXILA AMERICAN UNIVERSITY COLLEGE OF MEDICINE
Website: http://www.tauedu.org/

UNIVERSITY OF GUYANA FACULTY OF HEALTH SCIENCES
Website: http://uog.edu.gy/faculties/fhs/

UNIVERSITY OF THE WEST INDIES FACULTY OF MEDICINE – ST. AUGUSTINE
Website: http://sta.uwi.edu/fms/

WASHINGTON UNIVERSITY OF HEALTH AND SCIENCES
Website: http://www.wuhs.org/

XAVIER UNIVERSITY SCHOOL OF MEDICINE
Website: http://www.xusom.com

Other information was obtained from the following sources:

Alex' Illicit Guide to Medical School Admissions

American Association of Collegiate Registrar's and Admissions Officers (AACRAO)

American Board of Medical Specialties (ABMS)

American College of Surgeons (ACS)

American College Testing Program - Medical College Admissions Test

American Council on Education (ACE)

American Medical Association

American Medical Residency Certification Board (AMRCB®)

Association of American Medical Colleges (AAMC)

Association of Program Directors in Surgery Residency Clearinghouse

Canadian Resident Matching Service

Canadian Student Loan International Health Education Loan Program (TERI)

Caribbean Medical Schools - A Guide for Canadians

Clip Art provided by: www.worldatlas.com

Committee of Interns and Residents (CIR)

COTH Housestaff Survey

Council of Medical Specialty Societies (CMSS)

Department of Veterans Affairs

ECFMG Annual Report

ED-Invest Foreign Medical School Student Loan Program

Educational Commission for Foreign Medical Graduates (ECFMG®)

Educational Credential Evaluators, Inc.

Encarta Encyclopedia

Equifax

Experian

FAFSA

Federation of State Medical Boards of the United States (FSMB)

Federal Subsidized Stafford Loan Program

Federal Unsubsidized Stafford Loan Program (SLS)

Foundation for the Advancement of International Medical Education and Research (FAIMER®)

FREIDA

http://www.caribbeansupersite.com/bahamas/index.htm

http://www.islandconnoisseur.com/

http://www.valuemd.com

Institute of International Education

International Education Research Foundation, Inc.

International Medical Education Directory (IMED)

International Select Alternative Loan - Nation-wide Loan Program

Josef Silny & Associates, Inc. - International Education Consultants

Key Education Loan - MedAchiever Loan

Key Education Resources

MedCAP Alternative Loan for Health Professionals

Medical College Admission Test (MCAT®)

National Association of Credential Evaluation Services (NACES) member

National Board Medical Examiners (NBME)

NRMP® and ECFMG® Charting Outcomes in the Match for International Medical Graduates, 2014

National Resident Matching Program (NRMP®)

The Official Guide to Caribbean Medical Schools. (1997) Sarin, Salaish K. and Yalamanchi, Ravi K.

Philadelphia College of Osteopathic Medicine

Test of English as a Foreign Language (TOEFL®)

Trans Union Corporation

United States Medical Licensing Examination (USMLE®)

Veterans Benefits

Wikipedia

World Education Services, Inc.

World Health Organization (WHO)

www.aamc.org

http://www.caribbeanmedstudent.com/2009/09/the-accreditation-process-of-caribbean-medical-schools/

http://www.blog.trinityschoolofmedicine.org/blog-compare_Caribbean_-Medical_Schools/bid/105150/Where-can-I-Get-a-Residency-Get-Licensed-Trinity-School-of-Medicine-MD

Provincial and Territorial Student Assistance Offices in Canada

Newfoundland
Student Aid Division
Department of Education
Thompson Student Centre
P.O. Box 8700, 3rd floor
St. John's, Newfoundland A1B 4J6
1-888-657-0800
Phone: (709) 729-5849
Fax: (709) 729-2298
www.edu.gov.nf.ca/studentaid/

Nova Scotia
Student Assistance Office
Department of Education and
P.O. Box 2290, Halifax Central
Halifax, Nova Scotia B3J 3C8
Phone: (902) 424-8420
Fax: (902) 424-0540
1-800-565-8420 (in Nova Scotia)
Tel TDD: (902) 424-2058
http://www.ednet.ns.ca

Ontario
Student Affairs Branch
Ministry of Education/Training
189 Red River Road, 4th floor
P.O. Box 4500
Thunder Bay, Ontario P7B 6G9
Phone: (807) 343-7260
1-800-465-3013 (Ontario only)
1-800-465-3958 (TDD)
http://osap.gov.on.ca

Quebec
Direction générale de l'aide
financière aux étudiants
Ministère de l'éducation
1035, rue De La Chevrotière
Édifice Marie-Guyart, 22e étage
Québec (Québec) G1R 5A5
(418) 646-4505 (Québec)
(514) 864-4505 (Montréal)

New Brunswick
Student Services Branch
Department of Advanced Culture
Education and Labor
P.O. Box 6000, 548 York St.
Fredericton, N. B. E3B 5H1
Phone: (506) 453-2577
  1-800-667-5626
Fax: (506) 444-4333
www.gov.nb.ca/ael/stuaid/
  guide.htm

Manitoba
Student Financial Assistance
Dept. of Education and Training
409-1181 Portage Avenue
Winnipeg, Manitoba R3G 0T3
Phone: (204) 945-6321 or
(204) 945-2313 (out of province)
1-800-204-1684 (in Manitoba)
Fax: (204) 948-3421
http://www.edu.gov.mb.ca

Saskatchewan
Student Financial Assistance
Post-Secondary Education and Training
Room B21, 3085 Albert Street
Regina, Saskatchewan S4P 3V9
Phone: (306) 787-5620
Fax: (306) 787-7537
http://www.sasked.gov.sk.ca

British Columbia
Student Services Branch
Advanced Education, Training Skills and Technology
2nd Floor, 1106 Cook Street
Victoria, B.C. V8V 3Z9
Phone: (250) 387-6100

Northwest Territories
Student Financial Assistance
Department of Education, Culture Employment
P.O. Box 1320
Yellowknife, N.W.T X1A 2L9
Phone: (403) 873-7190 or
1-800-661-0793
Fax: (403) 873-0336 or
1-800-661-0893

Lower Mainland
P.O. Box 9173
Station Provincial government and
Victoria, B.C. V8W 9H7
1-800-561-1818 (in B.C.)
Fax: (250) 356-9455
http://www.est.gov.bc.ca

Alberta
Alberta Learner Assistance Division
http://www.aecd.gov.ab.ca/index.html

STUDENT DISCOUNTS AND ADVERTISING

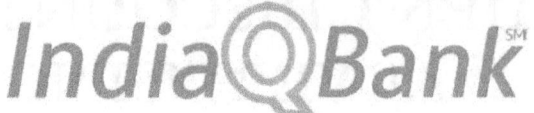

Prepare with Confidence!

Are you looking for quality, expert and accurate prep questions created by expert physicians? The American Medical Residency Certification Board® (AMRCB®) has partnered with IndiaQBank to offer an online study tool at a **25%** discount! IndiaQBank is an online study tool for helping you study and pass your AIPGMEE, FMGE, USMLE or JEE Mains boards.

If you identify an affiliation with the AMRCB® you will receive **25% off** the subscription that best fits your needs.

1. Access IndiaQBank question banks at www.indiaqbank.com
2. Sign-up by entering your name and email, choose a password and agree to terms and conditions.
3. Choose the test bank and the subscription that best fits your needs. IndiaQBank has multiple subscription terms to choose from.
4. When checking out, enter the code AMRCB for a **25%** discount off the purchase price.

- IndiaQBank is an online test preparation service for the Medical and Engineering exams of India.
- IndiaQBank features accuracy and expertise in question and case creation that will give you the very best studying preparation experience available for you to pass your Medical or Engineering Exam.
- Our MCQs and explanations have been created by expert physicians and engineers.
- The questions encountered on the qbank have been shown to mirror the exact questions encountered on the actual licensing exams.

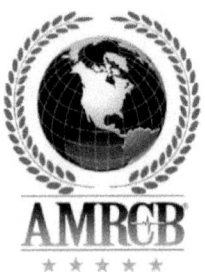
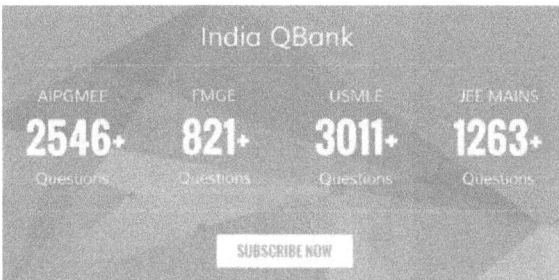

Central and South American Medical Schools - Caribbean Region

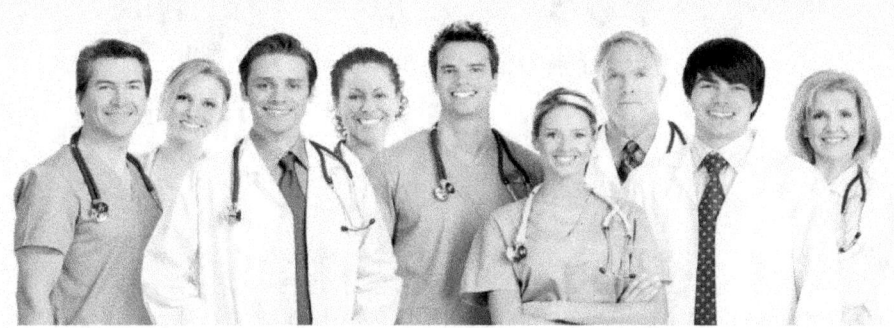

Enhance Physician Training Via the #1 Source for Specialty Medical Education

 WHAT IS BOARDVITALS?

BoardVitals™ is the largest and most used question bank for In-Service exams, Board Exams, Shelf Exams, and Physician Re-Certifications. We provide 20,000 questions, answers, and explanations targeted to over 20 medical and other healthcare specialities

BoardVitals TestBanks
Cardiology Child
Psychiatry
Dermatology Echo
Emergency Medicine ENT
Family Medicine GI
Internal Medicine
Neurology OBGYN
Pathology
Pediatrics
Psychiatry
Psychiatry Vignettes
Radiology
Surgery Shelf
Exams
USMLE Step 1
USMLE Step 2
USMLE Step 3

If you identify an affiliation with AMRCB using the links and steps below, you can purchase BoardVitals products at **10% off the individual price.**

1. Access BoardVitals products at:
   http://www.boardvitals.com/

2. Choose the test bank and the subscription term that best fits your needs: 1 Month, 3 Months or 6 Months

3. Enter your name and e-mail, choose a password and agree to the terms and conditions.

4. When checking out, enter in the code AMRCB for a 10% discount off the purchase price.

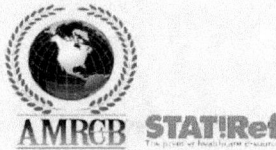

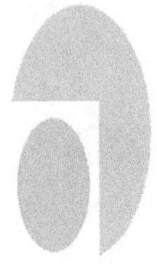
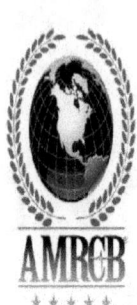

PCS
Practitioner Contracting Services

AMRCB is excited to partner with Practitioner Contracting Services to offer our clients an expert team to assist them in career planning. PCS offers over 30 years of combined experience in Health Law and now offers contract negotiations and career planning services to medical students, medical school, residents, fellows and practicing physicians. As a corporate partner with AMRCB, PCS offers a 20% discount to all AMRCB clients. The PCS fee is a flat fee, instead of the hourly fee you will find at most locations and companies. You can rest assured that no matter what comes your way, or how long it takes, your fee has been paid and it will cover everything.

For Medical Students: For our medical students PCS offers both Personal Statement review and Visa guidance. Personal statements are the first thing potential residency programs see; along with your CV and test scores. It is vital that students make a great first impression with their personal statements and are able to convey all the wonderful attributes they bring to the table. PCS can assist with personal statements in all stages of completion; from helping you get started, helping you draft a statement, knowing what to include, grammar and typographical editing and creative writing review and assistance.

In addition to personal statement review, PCS offers Visa guidance. For many international students the Visa process can be very complicated and confusing; but PCS helps to eliminate those concerns. PCS assists student as they maneuver what forms need to be filed with which governmental agencies, how the process will work and what to expect along the way.

For Residents and Fellows: For residents, fellows and practicing physicians PCS offers both Visa guidance and contract review and negotiation. Along with the Visa guidance services discussed above, PCS also can assist physicians as they receive employment contracts with their chosen practice. PCS will review each contract to ensure it offers the best salary, benefits, avoids pitfalls and problem terms and offers the best protection for the physician. From start to finish, all aspects of the negotiation is included in the PCS service fee.

www.Practitionercontractingservices.com or call 1-904-342-7390

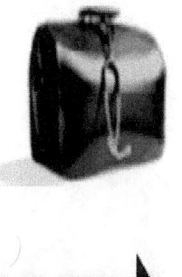

What is AttendingDr?

AttendingDr is a professional HIPAA-secure networking platform centered around the needs of physicians, built by practicing physicians. Whether you're a doctor or administrator in private practice or a hospital, AttendingDr serves to provide invaluable resources for your work and career. The platform includes a robust HIPAA-secure messaging, state-of-the-art patient referral system and scheduling software, Telemedicine platform, physicians' career center, credentialing system, and access to member benefits. Current member benefits include HIPAA-Insurance, discounts for malpractice, disability, and other insurance products, access to marketing assistance, and many other benefits. All this in a secure environment that will ensure privacy and security of your information.

AttendingDr was created with the collaboration of ideas from physicians, healthcare industry executives, and entrepreneurs. Join today or Inquire about our private white label solutions for your organization.

Visit **www.attendingdr.com** today!

Central and South American Medical Schools - Caribbean Region